Advances in
CNS Demyelinating Disorders

Indian Academy of Neurology

Advances in CNS Demyelinating Disorders

Editor-in-Chief

Debashish Chowdhury
DTCD MD(Medicine) DM(Neurology) FIAN FRCP(Edinburgh)
Commonwealth Fellow in Stroke Medicine(Edinburgh)
Director–Professor and Head
Department of Neurology
GB Pant Institute of Postgraduate Medical Education and Research
New Delhi, India

Editors

Rohit Bhatia MBBS MD DM DNB
Professor
Department of Neurology
AIIMS
New Delhi, India

Netravathi M MBBS DM
Professor
Department of Neurology
NIMHANS
Bengaluru, Karnataka, India

Bhawna Sharma MD DM FIAN
Senior Professor and Head
Department of Neurology
SMS Medical College
Jaipur, Rajasthan, India

Kamakshi Dhamija MD DM
PDF in CNS Demyelination
Senior Consultant
Department of Neurology
Max Super Speciality Hospital
Vaishali, Uttar Pradesh, India

Foreword

Bhim S Singhal

JAYPEE

JAYPEE BROTHERS MEDICAL PUBLISHERS

The Health Sciences Publisher

New Delhi | London

JAYPEE Jaypee Brothers Medical Publishers (P) Ltd

Headquarters
EMCA House
23/23-B, Ansari Road, Daryaganj
New Delhi 110 002, India
Landline: +91-11-23272143, +91-11-23272703
+91-11-23282021, +91-11-23245672
E-mail: jaypee@jaypeebrothers.com

Corporate Office
Jaypee Brothers Medical Publishers (P) Ltd.
4838/24, Ansari Road, Daryaganj
New Delhi 110 002, India
Phone: +91-11-43574357
Fax: +91-11-43574314
E-mail: jaypee@jaypeebrothers.com

Overseas Office
JP Medical Ltd.
83, Victoria Street, London
SW1H 0HW (UK)
Phone: +44-20 3170 8910
Fax: +44(0)20 3008 6180
E-mail: info@jpmedpub.com

Website: www.jaypeebrothers.com
Website: www.jaypeedigital.com

Inquiries for bulk sales may be solicited at: jaypee@jaypeebrothers.com

IAN Advances in CNS Demyelinating Disorders / ***Debashish Chowdhury, Rohit Bhatia, Netravathi M, Bhawna Sharma, Kamakshi Dhamija***

First Edition: 2025

ISBN: 978-93-6616-342-0

Printed in India

Dedication

This book is dedicated to our patients,
whose strength and resilience have helped us
understand the diseases on a deeper level.

Indian Academy of Neurology

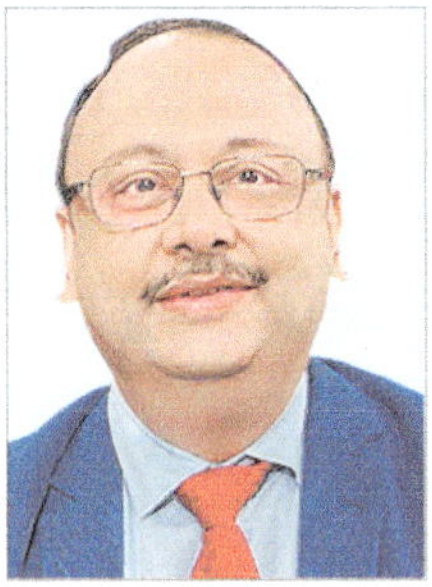

PRESIDENT
Debashish Chowdhury
New Delhi, India

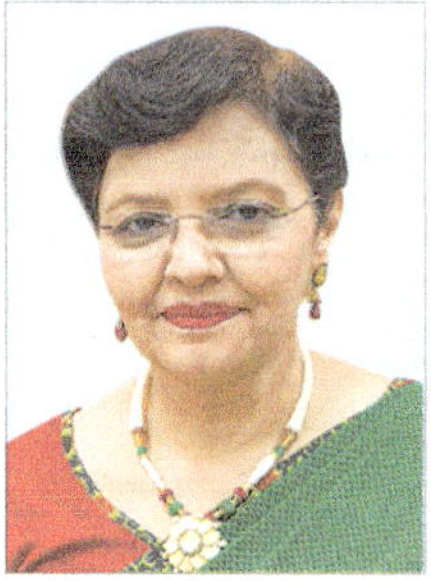

PRESIDENT-ELECT
Sangeeta Ravat
Mumbai, Maharashtra, India

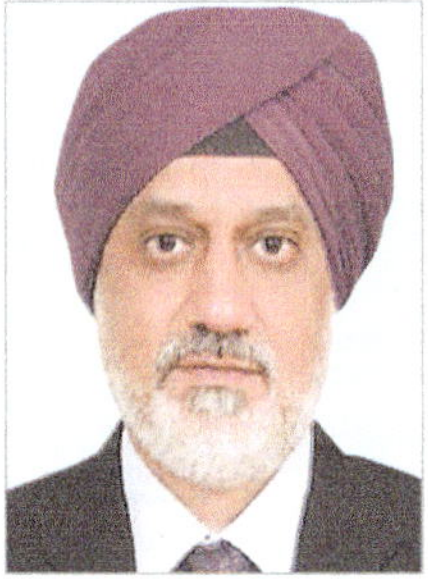

IMMEDIATE PAST PRESIDENT
Gagandeep Singh
Ludhiana, Punjab, India

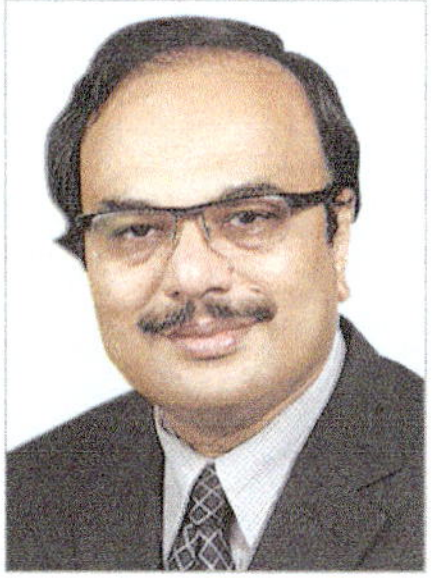

PAST PRESIDENT
Nirmal Surya
Mumbai, Maharashtra, India

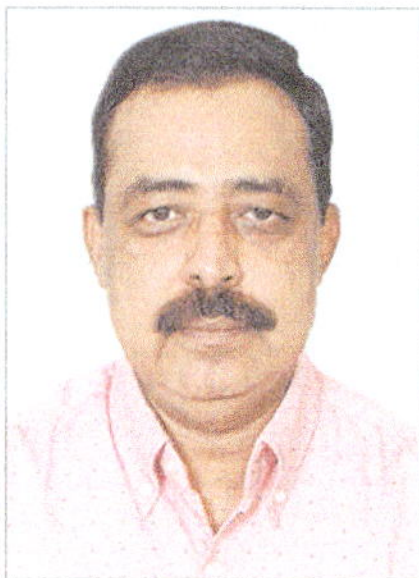

TREASURER
Achal Srivastava
New Delhi, India

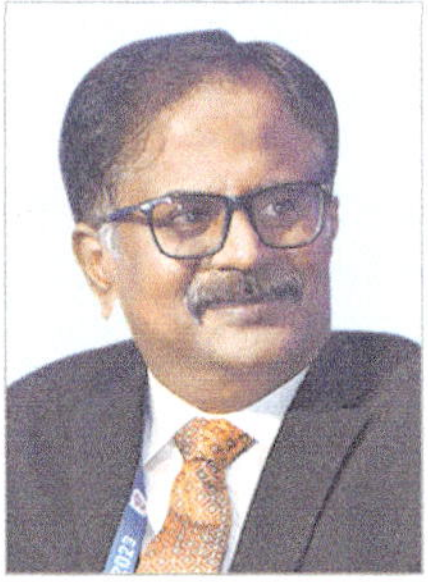

SECRETARY
U Meenakshisundaram
Chennai, Tamil Nadu, India

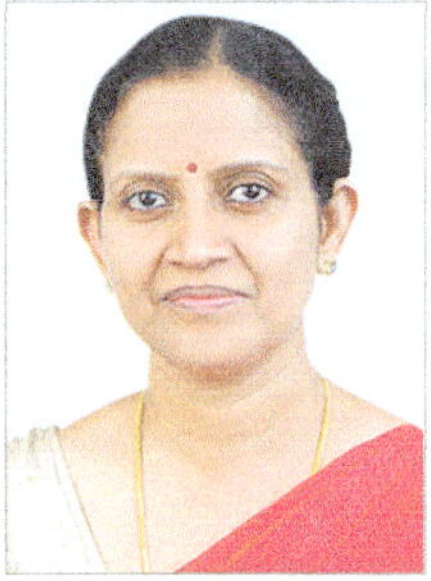

EDITOR, ANNALS OF IAN
PN Sylaja
Thiruvananthapuram, Kerala, India

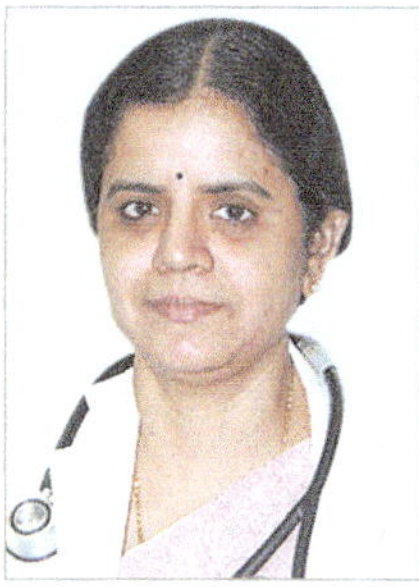

CME CONVENER
Sita Jayalakshmi
Hyderabad, Telangana, India

Executive Members

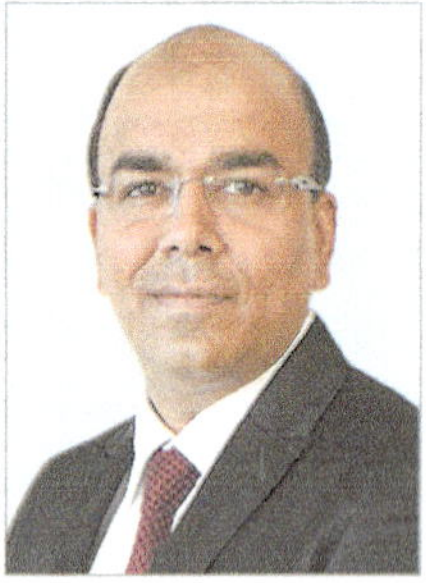

Arvind Sharma
Ahmedabad, Gujarat, India

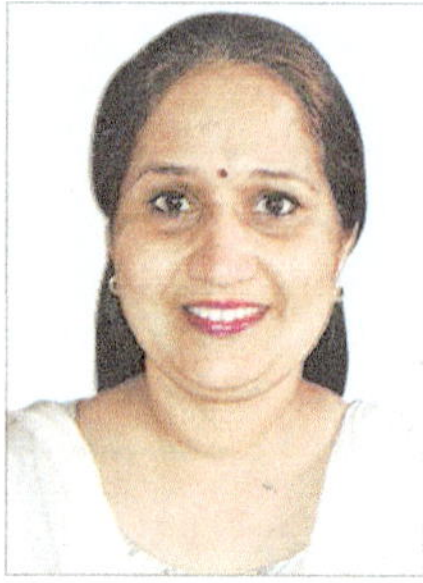

Bhawna Sharma
Jaipur, Rajasthan, India

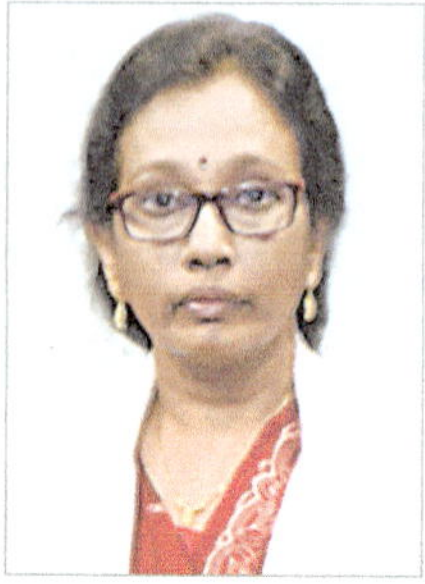

Atchayaram Nalini
Bengaluru, Karnataka, India

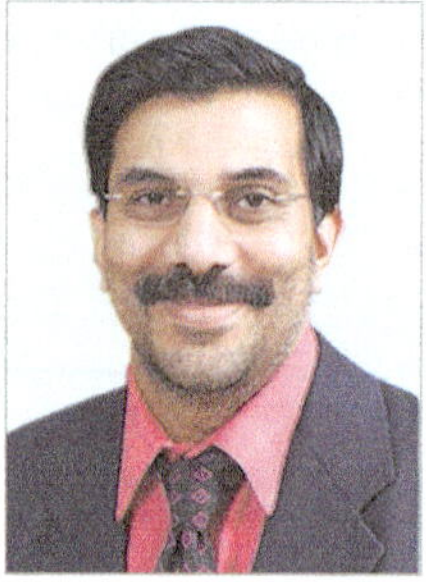

JOINT TREASURER
Pradeep VG
Kozhikode, Kerala, India

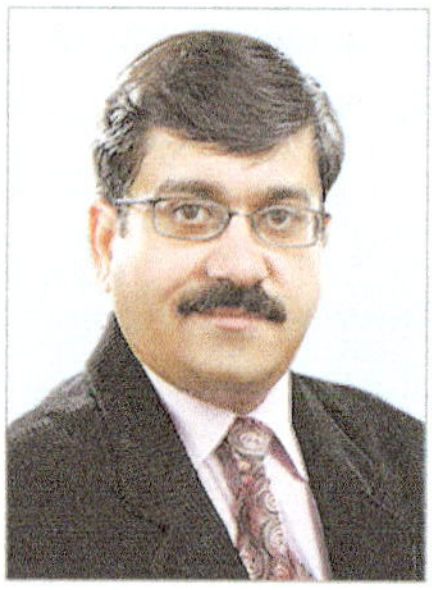

JOINT SECRETARY
Sumit Singh
Gurugram, Haryana, India

Contributors

Aditya Nayan MBBS MD DM
Senior Resident
PGIMER
Chandigarh, India

Areca Wangnoo MD DNB
Associate Consultant
Department of Neurology
PARAS Hospital
Gurugram, Haryana, India

AT Prabhakar MD(General Medicine) DM
Professor
Department of Neurology
Christian Medical College
Vellore
Vellore, Tamil Nadu, India

Ayush Agarwal MD DM DNB MNAMS Associate FAMS
Assistant Professor
Department of Neurology
AIIMS
New Delhi, India

Bhawna Sharma MD DM FIAN
Senior Professor and Head
Department of Neurology
SMS Medical College
Jaipur, Rajasthan, India

Dheeraj Khurana DM
Professor
PGIMER
Chandigarh, India

Dulari Gupta MD DM DNB(Neurology)
Associate Professor
Department of Neurology
Bharati Vidyapeeth (DU)
Medical College
Pune, Maharashtra, India

Jayanth SS MBBS MD DM
Postdoctoral Fellow in CNS
Demyelinating Disorders
National Institute of Mental
Health and Neurosciences
(NIMHANS)
Bengaluru, Karnataka, India

Jemini George DrNB
Postdoctoral Fellow
Department of Neurology
Sree Chitra Tirunal Institute
for Medical Sciences and
Technology
Thiruvananthapuram, Kerala,
India

Kamakshi Dhamija MD DM
PDF in CNS Demyelination
Senior Consultant
Department of Neurology
Max Super Speciality Hospital
Vaishali, Uttar Pradesh, India

Kandha Kumar UK MD DM
Associate Professor
Department of Pediatrics
AIIMS Jodhpur
Jodhpur, Rajasthan, India

Kshiteeja Jain MBBS MD DM
Postdoctoral Fellow in CNS
Demyelinating Disorders
National Institute of Mental
Health and Neurosciences
(NIMHANS)
Bengaluru, Karnataka, India

Lokesh Saini MD DM
Associate Professor
Department of Pediatrics
AIIMS Jodhpur
Jodhpur, Rajasthan, India

Madhuparna Paul DNB DM MRCP
Senior Consultant
Manipal Hospitals - Mukundapur
Kolkata, West Bengal, India

Minu George MD DM
Senior Consultant
Renai Medicity
Kochi, Kerala, India

Netravathi M MBBS DM
Professor
Department of Neurology
NIMHANS
Bengaluru, Karnataka, India

Padma Srivastava MD DM
Chairperson Neurology
PARAS Hospital
Gurugram, Haryana, India

Pritam Majumdar MD DM
Fellow in Neuroimmunology
St John's Medical College
Hospital
Bengaluru, Karnataka, India

Rohit Bhatia MBBS MD DM DNB
Professor
Department of Neurology
AIIMS
New Delhi, India

Siddharth Chand MBBS MD
DNB MRCP
Assistant Professor
PGIMER
Chandigarh, India

Sitla Prasad Pathak MBBS MD
DNB
Senior Consultant
Department of Neurology
Max Super Speciality Hospital
Vaishali, Uttar Pradesh, India

Soumya Sundaram DM
Additional Professor
Department of Neurology
Sree Chitra Tirunal Institute
for Medical Sciences and
Technology
Thiruvananthapuram, Kerala,
India

SP Gorthi MD DM FAAN SCE
Professor and Head
Department of Neurology
Bharati Vidyapeeth (DU)
Medical College
Pune, Maharashtra, India

Sruthi S Nair DM
Additional Professor
Department of Neurology
Sree Chitra Tirunal Institute
for Medical Sciences and
Technology
Thiruvananthapuram, Kerala,
India

Subhas Bhuin MD DM
Fellow in Neuroimmunology
Department of Neurology
PARAS Hospitals
Gurugram, Haryana, India

Sucharita Ray MBBS MD DM
PDF
Associate Professor
PGIMER
Chandigarh, India

**Suresh Kumar
Radhakrishnan** MD DM
Senior Consultant
Renai Medicity
Kochi, Kerala, India

Thomas Mathew MD DM FIAN
Professor of Neurology
St John's Medical College
Hospital
Bengaluru, Karnataka, India

Foreword

It is a privilege to have been asked to write the foreword for "*IAN Advances in CNS Demyelinating Disorders*". This book, edited by distinguished experts Drs Rohit Bhatia, Netravathi M, Bhawna Sharma, and Kamakshi Dhamija, brings together leading specialists to address key issues related to multiple sclerosis (MS) and other demyelinating disorders such as neuromyelitis optica (NMO) and myelin oligodendrocyte glycoprotein associated disorders (MOGAD).

The chapters provide comprehensive updates on the latest advances in the understanding, diagnosis, and management of MS, NMO, and MOGAD. In particular, the contributors discuss treatment approaches for relapsing- remitting MS, progressive MS, and the critical decision-making involved in switching therapies. Emerging therapeutic options are also thoroughly covered, giving readers a complete overview of the evolving landscape in the field.

An essential focus of the book is the guidance on reducing the risks associated with treatment. The authors detail preventive measures, including appropriate vaccination protocols, to minimize adverse drug effects. The editors have also ensured that the unique challenges of managing these disorders in pediatric patients, as well as during pregnancy and lactation, are addressed.

I commend the editors and contributors for producing a resource that will prove invaluable to practicing neurologists in India. As the prevalence of these disorders increases, it is crucial for neurologists to remain up to date with the latest diagnostic and therapeutic strategies to provide the best care for their patients.

Bhim S Singhal
MD FRCP DSc(Hon) FAMS
Director of Neurology
Bombay Hospital Institute of Medical Sciences
Mumbai, Maharashtra, India

Message from Editor-in-Chief

Dear Readers,

The Indian Academy of Neurology (IAN) has been at the forefront of neurology education and has a rich history of publications which rank high in terms of academic and scientific content. As President, it has been my pleasure to team up with my Executive Committee members, who are experts in various neurological subspecialties and high-quality and prolific authors with an impressive track record of publications, as editors and bring out a series of books which continue to hold high the tradition of IAN in terms of high-impact scientific content.

As Chief Editor of IAN "*Advances in CNS Demyelinating Disorders*", it is my pleasure to bring to you a book which sets the bar high for content—accurate, updated, and relevant—and at the same time presents it in a reader-friendly manner, which makes the book an ideal companion for everyone interested in the subject. I thank my colleagues and editors of this book, *Dr Rohit Bhatia, Dr Netravathi M, Dr Bhawna Sharma and Dr Kamakshi Dhamija*, for the shared vision of high-quality, focused content as well as excellent support rendered during the making of this book.

This has been our collective effort, and we sincerely hope that each of you will like reading this book as much as we loved bringing this out.

Debashish Chowdhury

Preface

The human body's most intricate system, the central nervous system (CNS), is in-charge of both sophisticated cognitive processes and the most fundamental movement abilities. At its core, the CNS depends on an efficient transmission of signals, a process facilitated by myelin—the insulating sheath that surrounds neurons. When this protective sheath is compromised, as seen in demyelinating disorders, the consequences can be profound and wide-ranging, affecting physical, emotional, and cognitive well-being.

As a field, the study of CNS demyelinating disorders is evolving rapidly. With advancements in imaging, biomarkers, and therapeutic interventions, the hope for more precise diagnoses and effective treatments is becoming a reality. Yet, these advancements also bring new questions and complexities and our understanding of these disorders is in a constant state of refinement with new therapeutic strategies offering both promise and caution.

The main focus of the book *"Advances in CNS Demyelinating Disorders"*, is to provide a comprehensive understanding of the management principles across the spectrum of CNS demyelinating disorders such as multiple sclerosis (MS), neuromyelitis optica spectrum disorder (NMOSD), myelin oligodendrocyte glycoprotein associated disease (MOGAD), and other seronegative entities. Each chapter delves into the multifaceted nature of these disorders, highlighting advances in research and clinical care while acknowledging the challenges that persist in their management.

This book is intended for clinicians and students who are striving to better understand and manage CNS demyelinating disorders. While significant progress has been made in improving outcomes for patients, much work remains to be done, particularly in areas of individualized treatment and long-term care strategies.

In compiling this volume, we are reminded of the resilience of individuals living with these conditions, as well as the dedication of the many professionals who support them. It is our hope that this book not only contributes to the growing body of knowledge but also inspires continued efforts to alleviate the burden of CNS demyelinating disorders, ultimately moving us closer to a future where these diseases can be effectively managed, if not entirely cured.

Debashish Chowdhury
Rohit Bhatia
Netravathi M
Bhawna Sharma
Kamakshi Dhamija

Acknowledgments

Writing this book has been a wonderful journey and we thank the Indian Academy of Neurology (IAN) to bestow upon us this opportunity to contribute to this important body of work. We thank all authors for contributing to the book. Their knowledge, dedication, and collaborative spirit have been essential to the creation of this book. We would also like to express our gratitude to Jaypee Brothers Medical Publishers for their unwavering support in bringing this book to life.

Debashish Chowdhury
Rohit Bhatia
Netravathi M
Bhawna Sharma
Kamakshi Dhamija

Contents

CHAPTER 1

Management of Relapses in Central Nervous System Demyelinating Disorders

SP Gorthi, Dulari Gupta

ABSTRACT

Central nervous system (CNS) demyelinating disorders are a group of disorders characterized by demyelination in the brain, spinal cord, and optic tracts. Patients can present with myriad symptoms including motor, sensory, cranial neuropathy, cerebellar, bowel, bladder, and sexual disturbances. With time, there is accumulation of disability with increasing number of relapses. In this chapter, the clinical presentation of relapses, appropriate investigations, and management are discussed. Treatment of relapses in CNS demyelinating diseases consists of high-dose steroids, adrenocorticotropic hormone (ACTH), plasmapheresis, immunoadsorption, and intravenous immunoglobulin.

Keywords: CNS demyelinating disorders, Acute relapses, Treatment, Multiple sclerosis, NMOSD, MOG disease.

INTRODUCTION

Central nervous system (CNS) demyelinating disorders are a group of disorders characterized by demyelination in the brain, spinal cord, and optic tracts. Patients can present with myriad symptoms including motor, sensory, cranial neuropathy, cerebellar, bowel, bladder, and sexual disturbances. Most of the disorders discussed here have a high chance of disease exacerbation in the same patient. In this chapter, we will review the investigations and treatment of acute relapses in CNS demyelinating disorders. Treatment of secondary demyelinating disorders will not be discussed in this chapter.

A *relapse/exacerbation/flare* of MS is defined as a monophasic clinical episode with patient-reported symptoms and objective findings typical of MS, reflecting a focal or multifocal inflammatory demyelinating event in the CNS, developing acutely or subacutely, with a duration of at least 24 hours, with or without recovery, and in the absence of fever or infection.[1] *Pseudorelapse* is a temporary worsening of preexisting multiple sclerosis (MS) symptoms due to increased temperature (Uhthoff phenomena), infection, medical illness, or metabolic disorders.

Not all attacks/relapses require treatment. Attacks characterized by only mild sensory symptoms such as paresthesia can be treated with symptomatic therapy alone.

A *relapsing episode of neuromyelitis optica spectrum disorder (NMOSD)* is defined as the emergence of new neurological symptoms and/or exacerbation of preexisting ones that persist for more than 24 hours, with or without new/enlarging or enhancing magnetic resonance imaging (MRI) lesions.[2]

TREATMENT OF ACUTE ATTACKS

High-dose Intravenous Corticosteroids

All acute demyelinating CNS disorders with significant functional disability and objective neurological impairment require treatment with high-dose steroids. Active or latent infection should be ruled out prior to starting corticosteroids (pneumonia and urinary tract infection).

Initial treatment consists of intravenous (IV) methylprednisolone 1,000 mg/day for 3–7 days with or without a short course of tapering oral steroids.[3,4] The duration of IV steroid therapy will be directed by the severity of the symptoms. Severe symptoms with significant disability will warrant 7 days of IV therapy, while minor symptoms might require only 3 days of IV therapy.

Oral prednisolone 1,250 mg/day or oral methylprednisolone 1,000 mg/day for 3–7 days with or without a short taper can also be given.[5] IV methylprednisolone has a higher peak concentration in the blood when compared with the same drug and dose given orally.[5] However, whether this peak drug concentration manifests in any clinical benefits is not known.

The mechanism of action of steroids includes reduction in CD4 count, reduction in cytokine release, stabilization of blood-brain barrier, and reduction in intracranial immunoglobulin G (IgG) synthesis.[3]

Side effects of high-dose steroids include hyperglycemia, hypertension, osteoporosis, neck of femur fractures, reduced bone mineral density, acute gastritis, psychiatric disturbances, myopathy, hypokalemia, and posterior subcapsular cataract. These side effects can be combated with oral hypoglycemic agents, antihypertensive medications, adequate calcium and vitamin D supplementation, proton pump inhibitors, and clonazepam and oral potassium supplementation.

Steroids in Acute Relapses of Multiple Sclerosis

Placebo-controlled trials: A meta-analysis of 377 subjects in six trials [four with methylprednisolone and two with adrenocorticotropic hormone (ACTH)] showed that both corticosteroids were effective in prevention of disease worsening in 5 weeks of onset of symptoms [odds ratio (OR) 0.37; 95% confidence interval (CI) 0.24–0.57].[6] There was no difference between the two steroids used. There was also no difference between short course (5 days) versus long course (15 days) steroid treatment.

Oral versus IV corticosteroids: Various studies comparing oral with IV corticosteroids did not find any difference in their efficacy in treatment of MS relapses.[7] In a meta-analysis of five randomized control trials, three trials studied change in Expanded Disability Status Scale (EDSS) at 4 weeks, while two trials looked at MRI changes at 4 weeks. There was no difference in the rate of subsequent relapses over the next 6 months either. The COPOUSEP trial was a multicenter, double-blinded, randomized control trial conducted in France.[8] 199 patients with relapsing-remitting MS were randomized in a 1:1 ratio to IV methylprednisolone or oral methylprednisolone 1,000 mg once a day for 3 days and primary outcome was reduction in EDSS by at least 1 point at 28 days follow-up. The study found that oral methylprednisolone (primary outcome achieved by 81% of participants) was noninferior to IV methylprednisolone (primary outcome achieved in 80% of participants) (absolute treatment difference 0.5%; 90% CI -9.5 to 10.4). An earlier randomized control trial from Britain studied 80 patients with MS treated with oral or IV methylprednisolone and compared change in EDSS at 1, 4, 12, and 24 weeks. This study also failed to find any significant benefit of IV methylprednisolone over oral methylprednisolone (mean difference in

EDSS was 0.07 points more in those taking oral methylprednisolone; 95% CI -0.46 to 0.60).[9] An Italian study compared 40 MS patients with 20 each receiving oral and IV methylprednisolone, the primary outcome was change in EDSS as well as reduction in gadolinium-enhancing lesions on MRI. They found that oral steroids were noninferior to IV steroids (mean difference in MRI lesion reduction -20%, 95% CI -48 to +5%).[10] It is to be concluded that there is class 1 evidence to treat acute relapses of MS with high-dose corticosteroids.

The *Optic Neuritis Treatment Trial (ONTT)* is a seminal trial published in the New England Journal of Medicine (NEJM) in 1992 that studied various treatment modalities including IV methylprednisolone, oral methylprednisolone, and oral placebo for optic neuritis.[11] In this trial, patients in the IV methylprednisolone group fared better at 6 months follow-up than the other two groups ($p = 0.001$). However, the difference in visual outcomes at 6 months was only marginal between the three groups. Oral prednisolone was not found to change the visual outcomes or hasten the rate of recovery. In fact, there were more cases of new optic neuritis on follow-up in the prednisolone group (IV methylprednisolone 13%, oral prednisolone 27%, and oral placebo 15%). The relative risk of new attacks of optic neuritis was 1.79 (95% CI 1.08–2.95) in the prednisolone group as compared to the placebo group. After the publication of this trial, the standard of care for optic neuritis has been IV methylprednisolone followed by a short taper of oral steroids over 2 weeks.

Steroids in Acute Relapses of Neuromyelitis Optica Spectrum Disorder

All attacks of NMOSD should be treated with high-dose corticosteroids as soon as possible. The faster the treatment is initiated, the higher the likelihood of remission. Unlike MS, patients with NMOSD are less likely to respond favorably to initial treatment with either high-dose steroids (84%) or plasmapheresis (8%). In a multicentric study from Germany, among 185 patients with a total of 871 attacks, 810 patients were treated with high-dose IV corticosteroids. Of these, 19% showed complete remission, 65% showed partial remission, and 16% showed no remission at all.[12] Following the acute therapy, low-dose maintenance oral steroids can be given for 3–6 months to prevent further attacks.[13] Thus, these patients are likely to require additional further treatment **(Flowchart 1)**.

Steroids in Acute Relapses of Myelin Oligodendrocyte Glycoprotein Antibody Disease

In patients with myelin oligodendrocyte glycoprotein antibody disease (MOGAD), acute attacks tend to be severe and mostly require early treatment to prevent long-term disability. Dose of IV corticosteroids is the same as that used in MS and NMOSD.[15,16] In adults, high-dose oral prednisolone 1,250 mg once a day for 5 days can be considered as an alternative to high-dose IV corticosteroids. Unlike NMOSD, MOGAD patients have good response to steroids often helping in establishing a diagnosis of MOGAD. A study of 122 attacks of MOGAD treatment with IV methylprednisolone resulted in complete recovery in 50%, partial recovery in 44%, and no recovery in 6% of patients. After the acute course of corticosteroids, some experts recommend oral steroids slowly tapered over a few months to reduce the recurrence of attacks. This will also act as a bridge between the acute steroid therapy and give time for steroid-sparing disease-modifying therapies to set into action. More studies are required about the role of oral tapering steroids since in patients with frequent relapses, this can lead to prolonged steroid treatment and associated side effects.

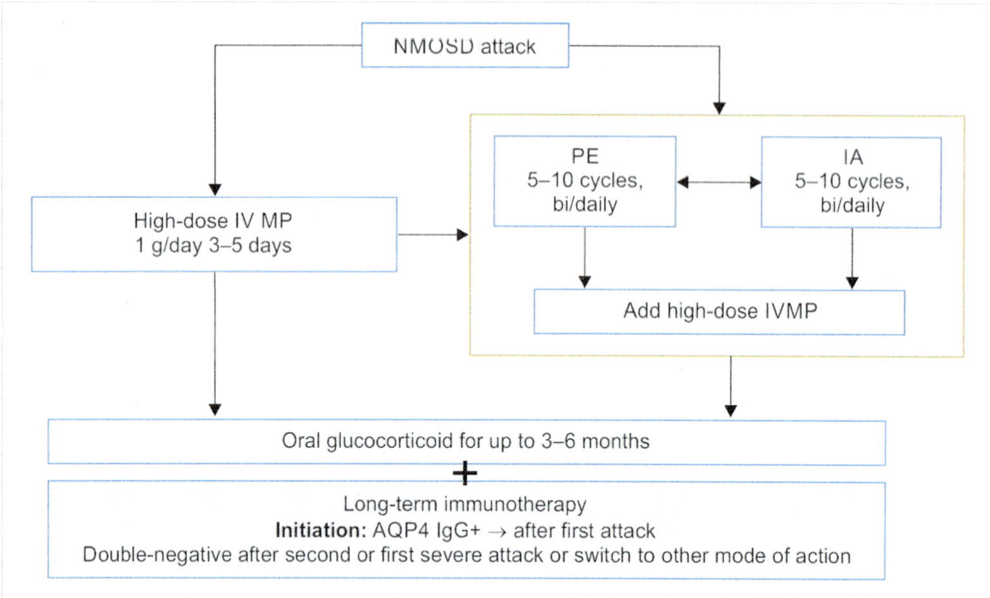

FLOWCHART 1: Treatment of NMOSD attack.[14]

(AQP4: aquaporin 4; IA: immunoadsorption; IgG: immunoglobulin G; IV: intravenous; MP: methylprednisolone; NMOSD: neuromyelitis optica spectrum disorder; PE: plasma exchange)

Adrenocorticotropic Hormone

Adrenocorticotropic hormone gel 80–120 U/day intramuscularly or subcutaneously for 1 or 2–3 weeks with or without a short taper.[17] It can be given as 80 U for 7 days, followed by 40 U for 4 days, and 20 U for 3 days. This drug and route are preferred by those patients who are unable to tolerate oral high-dose corticosteroids and prefer self-injection. However, ACTH gel is more expensive than IV or oral corticosteroids.

Plasmapheresis

Plasmapheresis can be used in cases which are resistant to high-dose corticosteroids or in those who show suboptimal response to steroids. Plasmapheresis is given in an alternate day schedule for five to seven cycles. Complications include catheter site infection, thrombosis, hypotension, and cardiac arrhythmias. Among 22 patients with CNS demyelination, patients treated with PLEX showed higher chances of neurological recovery (42% vs. 6%) in those who got placebo treatment.[18] In a randomized, double-blind, placebo-controlled trial among patients with severe CNS demyelination who failed to respond to high-dose corticosteroids, those treated with plasma exchange (PLEX) showed a good response (42.1% vs. 5.6%). Of these, 12 patients had MS, 4 had transverse myelitis, 1 had acute disseminated encephalomyelitis (ADEM), 1 had Marburg variant, and 2 had NMOSD.[19]

Plasmapheresis in Multiple Sclerosis

Plasmapheresis is indicated as second-line treatment in patients who have a poor response to first-line treatment with high-dose corticosteroids. It can also be used as first-line treatment in patients with large tumefactive demyelinating lesions with severe deficits or with optic neuritis with poor visual acuity (<20/400).[19] In a multicenter, double-blinded, randomized control trial,

116 patients with MS were treated with 11 sessions of PLEX compared with sham PLEX (placebo).[20] There was significant improvement in the PLEX group (64%) versus the placebo group (14%).

Plasmapheresis in Neuromyelitis Optica Spectrum Disorder

Few studies have shown that in severe attacks of NMOSD (defined as EDSS score ≥ 4 and/or visual acuity ≤ 20/200), early adjuvant plasmapheresis with high-dose IV corticosteroids has greater chances of improvement than steroids alone.[21] In the same study, those with isolated myelitis were more likely to respond to plasmapheresis or immunoadsorption than high-dose corticosteroids (*p*-value 0.037). Plasmapheresis is the treatment of choice for second-line treatment (34%) as well as for subsequent attacks (50%).[4,14] It has been found that in patients with severe attacks of NMOSD, if adjuvant plasmapheresis is started within 2 days of disease onset, the outcomes are better (40% complete recovery) than if it is started >7 days after disease onset (3.7% complete recovery).[21] Plasmapheresis can be considered the first-line treatment in cases where previous attacks were resistant to corticosteroids; previous attacks were responsive to plasmapheresis or severe myelitis.[14]

Plasmapheresis in Myelin Oligodendrocyte Glycoprotein Antibody Disease

In patients with MOGAD who are refractory to high-dose steroids, plasmapheresis is an alternative therapy which can be given in five to seven cycles on alternate days.[18]

Immunoadsorption

This is another type of apheresis that can selectively remove immunoglobulins from the circulation, unlike PLEX which nonselectively removes all plasma proteins. Unfortunately, this therapy is costly and is not readily available in many centers. One study compared 61 patients with corticosteroid-refractory MS who were treated with immunoadsorption or PLEX.[22] Both therapies showed an improvement in the MS functional score at 4 weeks, though immunoadsorption was slightly better than PLEX (MS functional composite score at 4 weeks was 86.7% in the immunoadsorption group compared to 76.7% in the PLEX group, *p*-value 0.034).

Intravenous Immunoglobulin

In patients where plasmapheresis is not feasible or not available, IV immunoglobulin at a dose of 2 g/kg over 5 days can be used, especially in children with MOGAD.[23] IV immunoglobulin was used in addition to IV methylprednisolone among 20 patients with NMOSD (31 events) and compared to IV methylprednisolone alone in 39 patients (72 events), improved disability after recurrent attacks ($p < 0.001$) but did not have any additional benefit in treating the first episodes of NMOSD.[24] In a meta-analysis, IV immunoglobulin has been found to reduce the relapse rate, reduce the emergence of new lesion, and present disease progression in MS.[25] It is not effective in secondary progressive MS.

CONCLUSION

There are multiple treatment options for acute relapses of CNS demyelinating disorders, with high-dose corticosteroids being the mainstay of treatment. Plasmapheresis is the second-line treatment but can be used as first-line treatment in conjugation with high-dose corticosteroids in severe attacks of NMOSD. Rituximab has been used in preventing relapses of CNS demyelinating disease, but it has no role in the treatment of acute relapses.[26]

REFERENCES

1. Thompson AJ, Banwell BL, Barkhof F, Carroll WM, Coetzee T, Comi G, et al. Diagnosis of multiple sclerosis: 2017 revisions of the McDonald criteria. Lancet Neurol. 2018;17(2):162-73.
2. Kessler RA, Mealy MA, Levy M. Early indicators of relapses vs. pseudorelapses in neuromyelitis optica spectrum disorder. Neurol Neuroimmunol Neuroinflamm. 2016;3(5):e269.
3. Frohman EM, Shah A, Eggenberger E, Metz L, Zivadinov R, Stüve O. Corticosteroids for Multiple Sclerosis: I. Application for Treating Exacerbations. Neurotherapeutics. 2007;4(4):618-26.
4. Sellner J, Boggild M, Clanet M, Hintzen RQ, Illes Z, Montalban X, et al. EFNS guidelines on diagnosis and management of neuromyelitis optica. Eur J Neurol. 2010;17(8):1019-32.
5. Morrow SA, Stoian CA, Dmitrovic J, Chan SC, Metz LM. The bioavailability of IV methylprednisolone and oral prednisone in multiple sclerosis. Neurology. 2004;63(6):1079-80.
6. Filippini G, Brusaferri F, Sibley WA, Citterio A, Ciucci G, Midgard R, et al. Corticosteroids or ACTH for acute exacerbations in multiple sclerosis. Cochrane Database Syst Rev. 2000;(4):CD001331.
7. Burton JM, O'Connor PW, Hohol M, Beyene J. Oral versus intravenous steroids for treatment of relapses in multiple sclerosis. Cochrane Database Syst Rev. 2012;12:CD006921.
8. Le Page E, Veillard D, Laplaud DA, Hamonic S, Wardi R, Lebrun C, et al. Oral versus intravenous high-dose methylprednisolone for treatment of relapses in patients with multiple sclerosis (COPOUSEP): a randomised, controlled, double-blind, non-inferiority trial. Lancet. 2015;386(9997): 974-81.
9. Barnes D, Hughes RA, Morris RW, Wade-Jones O, Brown P, Britton T, et al. Randomised trial of oral and intravenous methylprednisolone in acute relapses of multiple sclerosis. Lancet. 1997;349(9056):902-6.
10. Martinelli V, Rocca MA, Annovazzi P, Pulizzi A, Rodegher M, Martinelli Boneschi F, et al. A short-term randomized MRI study of high-dose oral vs intravenous methylprednisolone in MS. Neurology. 2009;73(22):1842-8.
11. Beck RW, Cleary PA, Anderson MM, Keltner JL, Shults WT, Kaufman DI, et al. A randomized, controlled trial of corticosteroids in the treatment of acute optic neuritis. The Optic Neuritis Study Group. N Engl J Med. 1992;326(9):581-8.
12. Kleiter I, Gahlen A, Borisow N, Fischer K, Wernecke KD, Wegner B, et al. Neuromyelitis optica: Evaluation of 871 attacks and 1,153 treatment courses. Ann Neurol. 2016;79(2):206-16.
13. Wang L, Du L, Li Q, Li F, Wang B, Zhao Y, et al. Neuromyelitis Optica Spectrum Disorder With Anti-Aquaporin-4 Antibody: Outcome Prediction Models. Front Immunol. 2022;13:873576.
14. Kümpfel T, Giglhuber K, Aktas O, Ayzenberg I, Bellmann-Strobl J, Häußler V, et al. Update on the diagnosis and treatment of neuromyelitis optica spectrum disorders (NMOSD) - revised recommendations of the Neuromyelitis Optica Study Group (NEMOS). Part II: Attack therapy and long-term management. J Neurol. 2024;271(1):141-76.
15. Sechi E, Cacciaguerra L, Chen JJ, Mariotto S, Fadda G, Dinoto A, et al. Myelin Oligodendrocyte Glycoprotein Antibody-Associated Disease (MOGAD): A Review of Clinical and MRI Features, Diagnosis, and Management. Front Neurol. 2022;13:885218.
16. Marignier R, Hacohen Y, Cobo-Calvo A, Pröbstel AK, Aktas O, Alexopoulos H, et al. Myelin-oligodendrocyte glycoprotein antibody-associated disease. Lancet Neurol. 2021;20(9): 762-72.
17. Thompson AJ, Kennard C, Swash M, Summers B, Yuill GM, Shepherd DI, et al. Relative efficacy of intravenous methylprednisolone and ACTH in the treatment of acute relapse in MS. Neurology. 1989;39(7):969-71.
18. Weinshenker BG, O'Brien PC, Petterson TM, Noseworthy JH, Lucchinetti CF, Dodick DW, et al. A randomized trial of plasma exchange in acute central nervous system inflammatory demyelinating disease. Ann Neurol. 1999;46(6): 878-86.
19. Cortese I, Chaudhry V, So YT, Cantor F, Cornblath DR, Rae-Grant A. Evidence-based guideline update: Plasmapheresis in neurologic disorders: report of the Therapeutics and Technology Assessment Subcommittee of the American Academy of Neurology. Neurology. 2011;76(3):294-300.
20. Weiner HL, Dau PC, Khatri BO, Petajan JH, Birnbaum G, McQuillen MP, et al. Double-blind study of true vs. sham plasma exchange in patients treated with immunosuppression for acute attacks of multiple sclerosis. Neurology. 1989;39(9):1143-9.

21. Bonnan M, Valentino R, Debeugny S, Merle H, Fergé JL, Mehdaoui H, et al. Short delay to initiate plasma exchange is the strongest predictor of outcome in severe attacks of NMO spectrum disorders. J Neurol Neurosurg Psychiatry. 2018;89(4):346-51.
22. Dorst J, Fangerau T, Taranu D, Eichele P, Dreyhaupt J, Michels S, et al. Safety and efficacy of immunoadsorption versus plasma exchange in steroid-refractory relapse of multiple sclerosis and clinically isolated syndrome: A randomised, parallel-group, controlled trial. EClinicalMedicine. 2019;16:98-106.
23. Bruijstens AL, Wendel EM, Lechner C, Bartels F, Finke C, Breu M, et al. E.U. paediatric MOG consortium consensus: Part 5 – Treatment of paediatric myelin oligodendrocyte glycoprotein antibody-associated disorders. Eur J Paediatr Neurol. 2020;29:41-53.
24. Lin J, Xue B, Zhu R, Pan J, Li J, Lin Y, et al. Intravenous immunoglobulin as the rescue treatment in NMOSD patients. Neurol Sci. 2021;42(9):3857-63.
25. Sørensen PS. Treatment of multiple sclerosis with intravenous immunoglobulin: review of clinical trials. Neurol Sci. 2003;24 Suppl 4:S227-30.
26. Chisari CG, Sgarlata E, Arena S, Toscano S, Luca M, Patti F. Rituximab for the treatment of multiple sclerosis: a review. J Neurol. 2022;269(1):159-83.

CHAPTER 2

Disease-modifying Agents in Relapsing–Remitting Multiple Sclerosis

Siddharth Chand, Aditya Nayan, Sucharita Ray, Dheeraj Khurana

ABSTRACT

The research for various drugs in the treatment armamentarium of multiple sclerosis (MS) is continually evolving. Various drugs have been developed for the treatment of different forms of MS which act at different spots in the pathogenetic process. In this chapter, we discuss the various drugs used in different forms of MS and analyze the evidence of use and the contraindications for the use of each of these agents.

Keywords: Multiple sclerosis, RRMS, Disease modifying therapy.

INTRODUCTION

Multiple sclerosis (MS) has a very heterogeneous clinical course. The disease is categorized into four types: (1) Relapsing-remitting MS (RRMS), (2) primary progressive MS (PPMS), (3) secondary progressive MS (SPMS), and (4) progressive-relapsing MS (PRMS).[1] Active forms of MS are also present. Approximately, 85% of MS patients have the typical RRMS, with distinct episodes of worsening symptoms (relapses) followed by periods of improvement or remission. The attacks must last for <24 hours and it is crucial to differentiate them from pseudorelapses or temporary worsening of MS symptoms caused by stress or infection, which are related to preexisting MS lesions and not due to new areas of demyelination.[2]

Over the past 20–30 years, extensive research has been done on the etiopathogenesis of MS, with a focus on T-cell and B-cell immunity. The knowledge has helped in the development and evaluation of various drugs targeting these pathways. There has been a significant expansion in the number of disease-modifying therapies (DMTs) for MS, focusing on different targets. The efficacy of these new agents is robustly supported by data from randomized controlled trials (RCTs) and meta-analyses. In this chapter, we focus on the various DMTs used in different forms of MS with special emphasis on agents that have become popular for the treatment of RRMS in the post-interferon (post-IFN) era.

CHOICE OF DISEASE-MODIFYING THERAPY

Selecting an appropriate DMT for an individual patient is a complex process that includes addressing various concerns. The following are the most prominent issues to address:

- *Patient concerns*: Each patient is a unique combination of discussion points spanning various domains, including lifestyle, occupation, activity levels, allergies, and personal goals. Careful consideration of each of these factors can help in making a choice of therapy that best aligns with their expectations and needs.
- *Drug efficacy*: The effectiveness of a DMT in reducing the frequency of relapses, delaying progression, and improving magnetic resonance imaging (MRI) outcomes is one of the most crucial factors in the decision-making process. Comparative efficacy data vis-à-vis other drugs, especially in evidence-backed settings are an ideal proposition. Many drugs are also chosen because of cost considerations, especially in resource-limited settings.[3]
- *Convenience of administration*: The mode of administration (oral, injectable, or infusion), frequency of dosing, and the required monitoring can significantly impact patient adherence and quality of life. Therapies that are easier to administer and require less frequent dosing are often preferred.
- *Cost benefit and efficacy*: The financial burden of DMTs is not just a concern for the price of procuring the drug itself but also includes the cost of administration, including infusion, travel, vaccinations, serological tests, travel to the site of administration, etc. Insurance coverage and availability of patient assistance programs are measures available to a select few. However, these issues often become the most important barriers to evidence-based decision-making in developing countries.[4]
- *Adverse effect profile*: The side effect profiles of DMTs vary, with some therapies associated with more severe or more frequent adverse effects. Patient tolerance for these side effects is key to choosing the appropriate treatment.
- *Pregnancy and other conditions*: For women of childbearing age, the safety of DMTs during pregnancy is a critical consideration. Some therapies may pose risks to the fetus, necessitating careful planning and consultation with healthcare providers.

Various study designs have been used in the study of individual drugs. Many of the newer therapies go into clinical trials after phase II trials are completed. Expert group meetings have cited the usage of innovative clinical designs, incorporation of biomarkers, and intermediate outcomes to advocate the appropriate drug for MS.[5] Today, the treatment landscape for MS continues to evolve with more than 18 immunomodulatory DMTs currently approved for use in the US and Europe **(Tables 1 and 2)**. These DMTs are designed to treat various forms of MS including clinically isolated syndrome (CIS), RRMS, PPMS, and SPMS.

Despite the progress made over the past decades, the search for the most efficacious, safe, affordable DMT continues. Ongoing research, including head-to-head trials and real-world studies, will further refine the understanding of how to best manage MS with the available therapies. While the expanding array of DMTs offers new opportunities for improved management of MS, choosing the right therapy requires a nuanced approach that considers individual patient factors and the latest clinical evidence.

In the management of RRMS, two main treatment strategies that are utilized are the tiered escalation approach using lower initial treatment efficacy (LITE) and the high-efficacy frontline treatment (HEFT).[6]

TABLE 1: Classification of approved disease-modifying therapies in multiple sclerosis.

Class of drug	Drug name
Anti-CD20 monoclonal antibodies	• Ofatumumab (subcutaneous) • Ocrelizumab (intravenous) • Ublituximab (intravenous)
Integrin receptor antagonist	Natalizumab (intravenous)
Sphingosine 1-phosphate (S1P) receptor modulators (oral administration)	• Fingolimod • Siponimod • Ozanimod • Ponesimod
Fumarates (oral administration)	• Dimethyl fumarate • Monomethyl fumarate • Diroximel fumarate
Interferons	• Interferon beta-1b (subcutaneous) • Interferon beta-1a (subcutaneous or intramuscular) • Pegylated interferon beta-1a (subcutaneous)
Other agents	• Alemtuzumab (intravenous) • Cladribine (oral) • Teriflunomide (oral) • Glatiramer acetate (subcutaneous)

TABLE 2: Summary of approved DMTs for MS in clinical practice.

Drug name	Brand name	Mechanism of action	Route of administration	Approved US indication	US FDA approval year
Infusion and monoclonal therapies:					
Ofatumumab	Kesimpta	Anti-CD20 mAb	Subcutaneous	RRMS aSPMS	2020
Ocrelizumab	Ocrevus	Anti-CD20 mAb	Intravenous	RRMS PPMS	2017
Alemtuzumab	Lemtrada	CD52-directed mAb	Intravenous	RRMS	2014
Natalizumab	Tysabri	Integrin receptor antagonist	Intravenous	RRMS	2004
Ublituximab	Briumvi	Anti-CD20 mAb	Intravenous	RRMS aSPMS	2022
Mitoxantrone	Novantrone	Synthetic antineoplastic anthracenedione	Intravenous	RRMS SPMS PPMS	2000

Continued

Continued

Drug name	Brand name	Mechanism of action	Route of administration	Approved US indication	US FDA approval year
Oral medications:					
Ponesimod	Ponvory	S1P receptor modulator	Oral	RRMS	2021
Ozanimod	Zeposia	S1P receptor modulator	Oral	RRMS SPMS	2020
Siponimod	Mayzent	S1P receptor modulator	Oral	RRMS aSPMS	2019
Cladribine	Mavenclad	Purine antimetabolite	Oral	RRMS SPMS	2019
Dimethyl fumarate	Tecfidera	Unknown	Oral	RRMS	2013
Monomethyl fumarate	Bafiertam	Unknown	Oral	RRMS	2013
Diroximel fumarate	Vumerity	Unknown	Oral	RRMS	2013
Teriflunomide	Aubagio	Pyrimidine synthesis inhibitor	Oral	RRMS	2012
Fingolimod	Gilenya	S1P receptor modulator	Oral	RRMS	2010
Injectable therapies:					
Glatiramer acetate	Generic Glatopa Copaxone	Unknown	Subcutaneous	RRMS	2017 2015 1996
Pegylated IFN-β-1a	Plegridy	Unknown	Intramuscular Subcutaneous	RRMS	2021 2014
IFN-β-1b	• Betaseron (US) • Betaferon (EU) • Extavia	Unknown	Subcutaneous	RRMS	1993 2009
IFN-β-1a	• Rebif • Avonex	Unknown	Subcutaneous Intramuscular		1998 1996

(aSPMS: active secondary progressive multiple sclerosis; CD: cluster determinant; EU: European Union, FDA: Food and Drug Administration; IFN-β: interferon beta; mAb: monoclonal antibody; RRMS: relapsing remitting multiple sclerosis; S1P: sphingosine 1-phosphate; SPMS: secondary progressive multiple sclerosis; US: United States)

The LITE approach consists of tiered escalation with initial treatment beginning with drugs of moderate effectiveness, often referred to as platform therapies.

These include:

- IFN [e.g., IFN-(IFN-β)]
- Glatiramer acetate (GA)
- Teriflunomide

- Fumarates [e.g., dimethyl fumarate (DMF)]

Patients are closely monitored for treatment response, focusing on disease activity and disability progression. If ongoing disease activity or progressive disability is observed, treatment is escalated to high-efficacy agents such as:

- Natalizumab
- Anti-CD20 monoclonal antibodies (e.g., ocrelizumab and rituximab)
- Alemtuzumab
- Sphingosine 1-phosphate (S1P) receptor modulators (e.g., fingolimod and siponimod)
- Cladribine

The HEFT approach starts with high-efficacy agents early in the disease course to potentially achieve better long-term outcomes and reduce the risk of irreversible disability.

The choice between the LITE and HEFT approaches depends on several factors, including disease severity, patient preference, and the risk-benefit profile of the available treatments. While the LITE approach prioritizes safety and gradual escalation, the HEFT strategy aims for aggressive early intervention with high-efficacy treatments to potentially alter the disease course more significantly.

Assessment of disease progression: Traditionally, the primary aim of DMT for MS has been to reduce relapse rates and manage inflammation. However, with the advent of HEFT, disease management has shifted toward achieving a new outcome metric called No Evidence of Disease Activity (NEDA). NEDA encompasses three key indicators of disease activity: (1) Absence of relapses, (2) no progression in disability, and (3) no new or expanding MRI lesions (including new T2 lesions or gadolinium-enhancing lesions, which might indicate subclinical relapses). Since NEDA-3 primarily addresses the inflammatory aspects of MS, brain volume loss (BVL) observed through MRI has been suggested as an additional measure to create NEDA-4, providing insight into the neurodegenerative aspects of the disease.

Recent evidence from studies has shown that patients on LITE do not achieve NEDA-4. Analysis of 694 patients from the Norwegian registry showed that patients on high-efficacy DMTs are significantly more likely to achieve NEDA-4 at both years 1 and 2 compared to those on moderate-efficacy therapies, with the initial choice of treatment being the most crucial factor. At the end of the first year, 68.0% of patients who began treatment with a high-efficacy DMT as their initial medication achieved NEDA, compared to 36.0% of those who started with a moderate-efficacy DMT. By the second year, 52.4% of the high-efficacy group reached NEDA, while only 19.4% of the moderate-efficacy group did.[7]

Natural history of MS has shown that the maximum chance of relapses and MRI activity are at the onset. Hence, drug choice, selection, and escalation with escalating immunotherapy constitute a therapeutic approach grounded in a reasoned decision-making process, whereby treatments with the most advantageous risk/benefit ratio are prioritized initially.[6] Here, we discuss in detail some of the commonly used oral and parenteral DMTs and newer drugs that have been approved for use.

Teriflunomide

Teriflunomide is an oral medication that is an active metabolite of leflunomide, a drug commonly used for rheumatoid arthritis. It works by inhibiting dihydroorotate dehydrogenase (DHODH), an important mitochondrial enzyme involved in the production of pyrimidines needed by rapidly dividing cells.[8] Oral bioavailability is 100%, with peak drug levels within a couple of hours after ingestion. In MS, teriflunomide decreases the activity of proliferating T- and

B-lymphocytes, thereby reducing overall inflammation. Unlike cytotoxic drugs, teriflunomide is cytostatic and does not affect hematopoietic cell lines because these cells use a DHODH-independent "salvage pathway" to produce necessary pyrimidines. Teriflunomide has complete oral bioavailability, with peak plasma levels reached within 1–2 hours after intake. It has been used as a DMT for relapsing forms of MS for over a decade. Two of the largest trials in teriflunomide were TEMSO and TOWER studies. These studies showed a slightly reduced sustained disability progression [20.2% vs. 27.3% in TEMSO and a hazard ratio (HR) of 0.68 in TOWER] compared to a placebo in RRMS patients.[8,9]

The biggest benefit of teriflunomide over the commonly prescribed DMF is reduced loss of brain volume in the former agent.[10] This effect was remarkable in the long-term extension study of the TEMSO study. The most reported side effects of teriflunomide were gastrointestinal disturbances, thinning of hair, increased liver enzymes, and cytopenia. These side effects were related to the dosage and rarely led to patients discontinuing the treatment.

Dimethyl Fumarate

Dimethyl fumarate is a dimethyl ester of fumaric acid which has been used in the treatment of psoriasis. The precise mechanism by which DMF benefits MS patients is complex and not yet fully understood. Treatment with DMF leads to reductions in both CD4+ and CD8+ T-cell populations, with CD8+ T-cells being more significantly affected, resulting in an increased CD4+/CD8+ ratio.

Two major phase III trials, DEFINE and CONFIRM, assessed the effectiveness of DMF in patients with RRMS over 2 years. In the DEFINE study, DMF was tested at two doses, 240 mg twice daily and 240 mg three times daily, against a placebo.[11] DMF led to significant reductions in the annualized relapse rate (ARR), with relative reductions of 53% for the twice-daily dose and 48% for the thrice-daily dose. Similarly, the CONFIRM study showed relative ARR reductions of 44% for twice daily and 51% for thrice daily compared to placebo.[12] Both studies also found that DMF significantly decreased the number of gadolinium-enhancing lesions and new or expanding T2-hyperintense lesions on MRI. The CONFIRM study included an active comparator, GA, but was not designed to determine if DMF was superior or noninferior to GA. Post hoc analyses indicated that DMF had a significantly greater effect on ARR, new or expanding T2-hyperintense lesions, and new T1-hypointense lesions compared to GA. The ENDORSE was a completed extension study of the DEFINE/CONFIRM trials that assessed the long-term safety and effectiveness of DMF in patients with RRMS. For patients continuously on DMF ($n = 501$), the ARR remained low at 0.143 [95% confidence interval (CI) 0.120–0.169]. In those who switched from placebo to DMF ($n = 249$), the ARR decreased after starting DMF and stayed low, with an ARR of 0.330 (95% CI 0.266–0.408) for the first 2 years and an overall ARR of 0.151 (95% CI 0.118–0.194) for the entire ENDORSE study. Over 10 years, 72% of patients on continuous DMF and 73% of those who switched from placebo to DMF did not experience confirmed disability worsening over 24 weeks.[13]

Anti-CD20 Immunoglobulin G1 Monoclonal Antibodies

Ocrelizumab

Ocrelizumab is a second-generation humanized monoclonal antibody acting against the CD20 antigen. It is approved for both RRMS and PPMS. Unlike rituximab, it is known to exert more antibody-dependent cellular cytotoxicity (ADCC) activity than complement-dependent cytotoxicity (CDC) activity.

The OPERA I and OPERA II trials were pivotal studies evaluating the efficacy and safety of ocrelizumab in treating RRMS.[14] The trials recruited 821 and 835 patients with RRMS to receive intravenous (IV) ocrelizumab at a dose of 600 mg every 24 weeks or subcutaneous (SC) IFN β-1a at a dose of 44 μg three times weekly for 96 weeks. The OPERA I trial demonstrated that ocrelizumab significantly reduced the ARR compared to IFN β-1a, with a reduction of 46.5% ($p < 0.001$). Additionally, ocrelizumab led to a greater decrease in the number of new or enlarging T2 lesions and gadolinium-enhancing lesions and was associated with improved disability outcomes. Like OPERA I, OPERA II showed that ocrelizumab significantly reduced the ARR by 47.3% compared to IFN β-1a ($p < 0.001$). It also showed reductions in new or enlarging T2 lesions and gadolinium-enhancing lesions, along with improved disability outcomes. Both trials concluded that ocrelizumab was effective in reducing relapses and slowing disease progression in relapsing MS, with a favorable safety profile. In the ORATORIO study involving patients with PPMS, 488 participants were randomly assigned to receive ocrelizumab, while 244 were assigned to a placebo. For most measures of 24-week confirmed disability progression, those who began treatment with ocrelizumab earlier had a lower proportion of disability progression compared to those who initially received a placebo. Specifically, the proportion of patients experiencing disability progression as measured by the expanded disability status scale (EDSS) was 51.7% in the ocrelizumab group versus 64.8% in the placebo group, showing a difference of 13.1% (95% CI 4.9–21.3; $p = 0.0018$).[15]

A recently published observational cohort study conducted between January 2015 and March 2021, analyzed patients of RRMS treated with ocrelizumab or rituximab, included in the MSBase registry and Danish Multiple Sclerosis Registry (DMSR). A total of 710 patients treated with ocrelizumab (414 MSBase, 296 DMSR) were matched with 186 patients treated with rituximab (110 MSBase, 76 DMSR).[16] The ARR ratio was higher in patients treated with rituximab than in those treated with ocrelizumab (ARR 0.20 vs. 0.09). The cumulative hazard of relapses was higher among patients treated with rituximab than those treated with ocrelizumab. However, no difference in the risk of disability accumulation was observed between groups. IV ocrelizumab is given in an initial regimen of two doses of 300 mg each, administered on day 0 and day 14. Following this, it is administered as a 600 mg dose every 6 months.

Real-world effectiveness data for ocrelizumab has been mostly favorable. This has caused ocrelizumab to be one of the most used agents in the treatment of both relapsing and progressive forms of MS. The effect size has reflected the results in the pivotal OPERA and ORATORIO trials and further studies in populations not adequately represented by the pivotal trials. The dosing frequency is an attractive option and overall, the outcomes seem to suggest that ocrelizumab is a favorable option for use in diverse populations for both relapsing and progressive forms of MS.[17]

Rituximab

Rituximab is a monoclonal antibody against the CD20 antigen in B lymphocytes. It results in depletion in B cells and it is known to exert a higher effect on CDC activity than ADCC activity. While rituximab is frequently utilized in the treatment of MS, it has not received FDA approval for this condition. However, it has recently been added to the list of essential medicines for MS by the World Health Organization (WHO).[18]

Initial efficacy data came from a phase-2, double-blind, RCT involving 104 patients with RRMS.[19] 69 patients were IV rituximab 1,000 mg on days 1 and 15, and 35 patients received a placebo. Compared to the patients who received a placebo, those treated with rituximab showed a significant reduction in the number of total gadolinium-enhancing lesions at weeks 12, 16, 20, and 24, as well as a decrease in new gadolinium-enhancing lesions over the same period. Additionally, the proportion of patients experiencing relapses in the rituximab group was significantly lower at week 24 (14.5% vs. 34.3%, $p = 0.02$) and week 48 (20.3% vs. 40.0%, $p = 0.04$) compared to the placebo group. A subsequent study of rituximab as an add-on injectable showed similar findings of a significant reduction in the number of gadolinium-enhancing brain lesions in follow-up.[20]

Despite the initial success in phase 2 trials, subsequent large-scale phase 3 trials have not been done and the focus has of late shifted to ocrelizumab and ofatumumab. However, rituximab continued to be used as an off-label drug for MS in many centers.

Retrospective analysis from two Swedish cohorts showed that the annual discontinuation rate for rituximab because of clinical relapses and/or neuroradiologic disease activity was significantly lower for rituximab compared with injectable DMTs and DMF.[21] In another European observational study involving 453 MS patients, 82 were treated with rituximab. During the study, only three relapses were reported, and 59 patients (75.6%) did not experience any NEDA-3 by the end of follow-up. The time to evidence of disease activity was comparable between patients treated with rituximab and those treated with natalizumab, with a HR of 1.64 (95% CI 0.46–5.85; $p = 0.44$).[22]

Ofatumumab

Ofatumumab is a fully human, anti-CD20 monoclonal antibody. Patients can self-administer it subcutaneously. Ofatumumab exhibits more potent CDC activity than rituximab. It binds more firmly to CD20 and has a slower dissociation rate from CD20 compared to rituximab. Additionally, ofatumumab demonstrates greater effectiveness in C3b deposition and causes more pronounced cell lysis, including plasma membrane bulging and streamer formation, in various B cell lines than rituximab. Furthermore, ofatumumab is less reliant on the density of CD20 on the surface of target cells compared to rituximab.

The ASCLEPIOS I and ASCLEPIOS II trials were two double-blind, double-dummy, phase 3 trials, where patients of RRMS were randomly assigned to receive SC ofatumumab (20 mg every 4 weeks after 20 mg loading doses at days 1, 7, and 14) or oral teriflunomide (14 mg daily) for up to 30 months.[23] In the ASCLEPIOS I trial, the ARR was 0.11 for those treated with ofatumumab and 0.22 for those receiving teriflunomide (difference –0.11; $p < 0.001$). Similarly, in the ASCLEPIOS II trial, the rates were 0.10 for the ofatumumab group and 0.25 for the teriflunomide group (difference –0.15; $p < 0.001$). In the pooled analysis, the ofatumumab group had fewer gadolinium-enhancing lesions per T1-weighted MRI scan, a lower annualized rate of lesions on T2-weighted MRI and reduced serum neurofilament light chain levels.[23]

A network meta-analysis of 30 trials highlighted that ofatumumab generally performed better in controlling disease activity compared to therapies such as IFN β, GA, and teriflunomide.[24] However, it was less effective compared to some higher-efficacy treatments such as natalizumab and fingolimod.

Ublituximab

Ublituximab is a chimeric anti-CD20 antibody glycoengineered to exhibit potent B-cell depletion. Like ocrelizumab, it exhibits more ADCC activity. It binds to a distinct segment of the large extracellular loop, as well as to a region that overlaps with the epitopes targeted by rituximab and ocrelizumab.

In phase 3, double-blind, double-dummy ULTIMATE I and II trials, participants with

RRMS were randomized to receive either IV ublituximab (150 mg on day 1, followed by 450 mg on day 15 and at weeks 24, 48, and 72) with oral placebo, or oral teriflunomide (14 mg daily) with IV placebo. In both trials, the ARR and rate of gadolinium-enhanced MRI lesions were significantly lower in patients treated with ublituximab as compared to the teriflunomide group.[25]

Sphingosine 1 Receptor Modulators

Sphingosine 1-phosphate receptor modulators are a class of DMTs targeting S1P receptors. These modulators bind to S1P receptors on lymphocytes, leading to their internalization and degradation, which prevents lymphocytes from leaving lymphoid tissues.[26]

Fingolimod

Fingolimod, the first approved S1P receptor modulator for treating RRMS, has been shown in clinical trials to reduce relapse rates, the number of gadolinium-enhancing lesions, new or enlarging T2 lesions, and BVL on MRI while also slowing disability progression. It is also the first oral agent used for the treatment of RRMS. The FREEDOMS and TRANSFORMS study demonstrated the efficacy of fingolimod in patients of RRMS when compared to placebo and IFN-βa, respectively.[27,28] The recommended dose is 0.5 mg once daily. Being a nonselective S1P receptor modulator, fingolimod has been associated with arrhythmia, heart block, macula edema, deranged liver enzymes, etc.[27-29] The trials and the extension studies showed a disproportionately increased risk of Varicella zoster virus.[30] Hence, it is advisable to do a complete blood count, liver function test, electrocardiogram, ophthalmology examination, and varicella serology (if negative, varicella vaccination) before starting fingolimod. One of the biggest concerns in the use of fingolimod is safety concerns in pregnancy. Studies have shown that IFN does not interfere with mean birth weight, risk of preterm birth, or other adverse pregnancy outcomes.[31] In comparison, fingolimod has genuine concerns with use in pregnancy.[32]

Ozanimod

Ozanimod is an oral selective S1P receptor modulator that specifically targets the S1PR1 and S1PR5 receptor subtypes. The RADIANCE trial (phase 2/3) and SUNBEAM trial (phase 3) compared the efficacy of 0.5/1 mg ozanimod with placebo and IFN-β, respectively.[33,34] The DAYBREAK trial was an open-label extension.[35] Ozanimod was significantly associated with a reduction in the ARR during the treatment period. It also resulted in fewer gadolinium-enhancing lesions by the end of the trial compared to the control. Additionally, patients treated with ozanimod had a lower number of new or enlarging T2 lesions over the treatment period compared to those in the control group.

Ponesimod

Ponesimod is an orally administered, highly selective modulator of S1P receptor 1 and has no active metabolites, which minimizes the potential for drug-drug interactions. It rapidly and dose-dependently reduces peripheral blood lymphocyte counts by preventing their exit from lymphoid organs. The quick elimination of ponesimod and the reversibility of its effects on lymphocyte levels enable a swift restoration of normal immune function, which could be advantageous for safety during pregnancy planning, serious infections, or vaccinations. In a randomized, placebo-controlled, dose-finding phase 2 study in patients with relapsing MS, the 20 mg dose of ponesimod significantly decreased both the cumulative number of new gadolinium-enhancing T1 lesions and new or enlarging T2 lesions compared to placebo.[36]

The OPTIMUM study evaluated the efficacy and safety of ponesimod in patients with RRMS. It was a double-blind, active comparator study; patients were randomized to receive either 20 mg once-daily ponesimod or 14 mg once-daily teriflunomide. In the study, ponesimod demonstrated a 30.5% relative reduction in the ARR compared to teriflunomide. The odds ratio for achieving NEDA-3 was 1.70, highlighting a greater likelihood of achieving this outcome compared to teriflunomide.

Siponimod

Siponimod (Mayzent®) is a next-generation, selective S1P receptor 1 and 5 modulators. It has been tried in RRMS but is approved in several countries for the treatment of SPMS.

The BOLD study was a phase 2, adaptive, dose-ranging study with two cohorts having various doses of siponimod and placebo cohort 1 containing drug doses 10, 2, 0.5 mg, or placebo in 1:1:1:1 randomization and cohort 2 containing siponimod 1.25, 0.25 mg, or placebo once daily for 3 months in a 4:4:1. This study showed adverse effects in patients treated with siponimod for 6 months versus 3 months in various drug doses. The results of a meta-analysis of siponimod showed uncertain confidence in the capacity of 2 mg siponimod to reduce the ARR as compared to placebo. Headache, back pain, bradycardia, infections, and a rise in liver function tests were some of the common side effects.[37,38]

Alemtuzumab

Alemtuzumab is a humanized monoclonal antibody that targets CD52 on lymphocytes and monocytes. It works by depleting T- and B-cells through mechanisms involving ADCC and complement-mediated lysis. The CARE-MS I trial was designed to evaluate the efficacy and safety of first-line alemtuzumab compared to IFN β-1a in a phase 3 setting. In this trial, 75 patients (40%) in the IFN β-1a group experienced relapses (totaling 122 events), whereas 82 patients (22%) in the alemtuzumab group experienced relapses (totaling 119 events). The rate ratio for relapse was 0.45 (95% CI 0.32–0.63; $p < 0.0001$), indicating a 54.9% improvement with alemtuzumab.[39]

The CARE-MS II, on the other hand, focused on assessing alemtuzumab's efficacy and safety in patients who had relapsed despite receiving first-line treatment. In this study, 104 patients (51%) in the IFN β-1a group had relapses (totaling 201 events), compared to 147 patients (35%) in the alemtuzumab group (236 events). The rate ratio was 0.51 (95% CI 0.39–0.65; $p < 0.0001$), showing a 49.4% improvement with alemtuzumab. Additionally, 94 patients (47%) in the IFN β-1a group were relapse free at 2 years, while 278 patients (65%) in the alemtuzumab group were relapse free at the same time point ($p < 0.0001$).[40]

In a post hoc analysis of the combined CARE-MS data, the ARR for patients on alemtuzumab was 0.27 in the first 2 years and 0.16 in years 3–9. Over 9 years, 62% of these patients were free from 6-month confirmed disability worsening, 50% experienced 6-month confirmed disability improvement, and the median cumulative brain volume change was a decrease of 2.15%.[41] Infusion-related reactions are the most common adverse effects which have been in the case of alemtuzumab.

Cladribine

Cladribine functions by interfering with cellular metabolism, inhibiting deoxyribonucleic acid (DNA) synthesis and repair, and leading to cell apoptosis. In the RCT CLARITY, 1,326 patients of RRMS were randomly assigned in equal proportions to receive either one of two cumulative doses of cladribine tablets (3.5 or 5.25 mg/kg of body weight) or a matching placebo. The treatment was administered in two or four short courses during the first 48 weeks, followed by two additional short courses starting at weeks 48 and 52, totaling 8–20 days/year. Patients receiving cladribine tablets (both doses) had a significantly lower ARR compared to the placebo group (0.14 and 0.15 vs. 0.33; $p < 0.001$ for both comparisons) and a higher relapse-free rate (79.7% and 78.9% vs. 60.9%; $p < 0.001$ for both comparisons).[42] Recently, real-world experience was reported from the DMSR, which included prospectively enrolled cases from December, 2017 to June, 2021. Among the 268 patients who began treatment with cladribine tablets—comprising 89 men and 179 women with a median age of 40 years—there was a notable decrease in the ARR. Before starting cladribine, the ARR was 0.67 [95% CI (0.56, 0.79)], but it dropped to 0.11 [95% CI (0.08, 0.15)] during the first 2 years after initiating cladribine, representing an 84.8% reduction.[43] Headache and lymphopenia are the most commonly reported side effects.

DRUGS UNDER DEVELOPMENT

Bruton's tyrosine kinase (BTK) is an intracellular signaling molecule crucial for B-cell function and is present in various hematopoietic cells, excluding natural killer cells and mature plasma cells. It plays a key role in B-cell maturation, survival, and activation, as well as in cytokine production and T-cell stimulation. In patients with RRMS and SPMS, memory B-cells show elevated levels of phosphorylated BTK compared to healthy controls, indicating increased BTK activation. To address this, several BTK inhibitors are being tested for their safety and effectiveness in MS: Evobrutinib, fenebrutinib, remibrutinib, and tolebrutinib are in phase III trials, while orelabrutinib is in a phase II trial. These inhibitors aim to modulate BTK activity and potentially improve MS outcomes.[44]

PEDIATRIC MULTIPLE SCLEROSIS

Fingolimod was the first oral DMT approved by the Food and Drug Administration (FDA) for use in the pediatric age group. In the PARADIGMS trial, fingolimod showed significant superiority over IFN β-1a in reducing both clinical and MRI activity in pediatric MS patients, with an associated improvement in quality of life, though there was a slightly higher rate of serious adverse events.[45] Additionally, teriflunomide and DMF have been approved by the FDA and European Medicines Agency (EMA) for pediatric MS following positive results in the TERIKIDS and CONNECT trials, respectively, which demonstrated their efficacy and safety in children with relapsing forms of MS.[46,47]

CONCLUSION

Disease-modifying therapies have significantly advanced the management of MS and RRMS, offering a range of options that effectively reduce relapse rates and slow disease progression. The evolution of treatment goals toward achieving NEDA underscores a shift toward more comprehensive management strategies, aiming not just to control symptoms but to minimize long-term disability. Clinical trials and observational studies have demonstrated that various DMTs, including newer agents, can markedly impact disease activity and improve patient outcomes. As our understanding of MS continues to grow, ongoing research and the development of new therapies will be crucial in enhancing treatment efficacy and optimizing patient care in RRMS.

REFERENCES

1. Jacques FH. Defining the clinical course of multiple sclerosis: The 2013 revisions. Neurology. 2015;84(9):963.
2. Green AJ. Understanding pseudo. Neurology. 2009;72(19):1626-7.
3. Alvarez E, Nair KV, Tan H, Rathi K, Gabler NB, Maiese EM, et al. Real-world cost of care and site of care in patients with multiple sclerosis initiating infused disease-modifying therapies. J Med Econ. 2023;26(1):494-502.
4. Nicholas J, Halpern R, Ziehn M, Peterson-Brandt J, Leszko M, Deshpande C. Real-world cost of treatment for multiple sclerosis patients initiating and receiving infused disease-modifying therapies per recommended label in the United States. J Med Econ. 2020;23(8):885-93.
5. Marrie RA, Sormani MP, Apap Mangion S, Bovis F, Cheung WY, Cutter GR, et al. Improving the efficiency of clinical trials in multiple sclerosis. Mult Scler J. 2023;29(9):1136-48.
6. Selmaj K, Cree BAC, Barnett M, Thompson A, Hartung HP. Multiple sclerosis: time for early treatment with high-efficacy drugs. J Neurol. 2024;271(1):105-15.
7. Simonsen CS, Flemmen HØ, Broch L, Brunborg C, Berg-Hansen P, Moen SM, et al. Early High Efficacy Treatment in Multiple Sclerosis Is the Best Predictor of Future Disease Activity Over 1 and 2 Years in a Norwegian Population-Based Registry. Front Neurol. 2021;12:693017.
8. Oh J, O'Connor PW. Teriflunomide. Neurol Clin Pract. 2013;3(3):254-60.
9. Confavreux C, O'Connor P, Comi G, Freedman MS, Miller AE, Olsson TP, et al. Oral teriflunomide for patients with relapsing multiple sclerosis (TOWER): a randomised, double-blind, placebo-controlled, phase 3 trial. Lancet Neurol. 2014;13(3):247-56.
10. Sprenger T, Kappos L, Radue EW, Gaetano L, Mueller-Lenke N, Wuerfel J, et al. Association of brain volume loss and long-term disability outcomes in patients with multiple sclerosis treated with teriflunomide. Mult Scler J. 2020;26(10):1207-16.
11. Gold R, Kappos L, Arnold DL, Bar-Or A, Giovannoni G, Selmaj K, et al. Placebo-Controlled Phase 3 Study of Oral BG-12 for Relapsing Multiple Sclerosis. N Engl J Med. 2012;367(12):1098-107.
12. Fox RJ, Miller DH, Phillips JT, Hutchinson M, Havrdova E, Kita M, et al. Placebo-Controlled Phase 3 Study of Oral BG-12 or Glatiramer in Multiple Sclerosis. N Engl J Med. 2012;367(12):1087-97.
13. Amezcua L, Mao-Draayer Y, Vargas WS, Farber R, Schaefer S, Branco F, et al. Efficacy of Dimethyl Fumarate in Young Adults with Relapsing-Remitting Multiple Sclerosis: Analysis of the DEFINE, CONFIRM, and ENDORSE Studies. Neurol Ther. 2023;12(3):883-97.
14. Hauser SL, Bar-Or A, Comi G, Giovannoni G, Hartung HP, Hemmer B, et al. Ocrelizumab versus Interferon Beta-1a in Relapsing Multiple Sclerosis. N Engl J Med. 2017;376(3):221-34.
15. Wolinsky JS, Arnold DL, Brochet B, Hartung HP, Montalban X, Naismith RT, et al. Long-term follow-up from the ORATORIO trial of ocrelizumab for primary progressive multiple sclerosis: a post-hoc analysis from the ongoing open-label extension of the randomised, placebo-controlled, phase 3 trial. Lancet Neurol. 2020;19(12):998-1009.
16. Roos I, Hughes S, McDonnell G, Malpas CB, Sharmin S, Boz C, et al. Rituximab vs Ocrelizumab in Relapsing-Remitting Multiple Sclerosis. JAMA Neurol. 2023;80(8):789.
17. Alcalá C, Quintanilla-Bordás C, Gascón F, Sempere ÁP, Navarro L, Carcelén-Gadea M, et al. Effectiveness of rituximab vs. ocrelizumab for the treatment of primary progressive multiple sclerosis: a real-world observational study. J Neurol. 2022;269(7):3676-81.
18. World Health Organization. (2023). The selection and use of essential medicines. [online] Available from https://iris.who.int/bitstream/handle/10665/371291/WHO-MHP-HPS-EML-2023.01-eng.pdf?sequence=1 [Last accessed September, 2024].
19. Hauser SL, Arnold DL, Fox RJ, Sarkar N, Smith CH. B-Cell Depletion with Rituximab in Relapsing–Remitting Multiple Sclerosis. N Engl J Med. 2008;358(7):676-88.
20. Naismith RT, Piccio L, Lyons JA, Lauber J, Tutlam NT, Parks BJ, et al. Rituximab add-on therapy for breakthrough relapsing multiple sclerosis: A 52-week phase II trial. Neurology. 2010;74(23):1860-7.
21. Granqvist M, Boremalm M, Poorghobad A, Svenningsson A, Salzer J, Frisell T, et al. Comparative Effectiveness of Rituximab and Other Initial Treatment Choices for Multiple Sclerosis. JAMA Neurol. 2018;75(3):320-7.
22. Scotti B, Disanto G, Sacco R, Guigli M, Zecca C, Gobbi C. Effectiveness and safety of Rituximab in multiple sclerosis: an observational study from Southern Switzerland. PLoS One. 2018; 13(5):e0197415.

23. Hauser SL, Bar-Or A, Cohen JA, Comi G, Correale J, Coyle PK, et al. Ofatumumab versus Teriflunomide in Multiple Sclerosis. N Engl J Med. 2020;383(6):546-57.
24. Samjoo IA, Worthington E, Drudge C, Zhao M, Cameron C, Häring DA, et al. Comparison of ofatumumab and other disease-modifying therapies for relapsing multiple sclerosis: a network meta-analysis. J Comp Eff Res. 2020;9(18):1255-74.
25. Steinman L, Fox E, Hartung HP, Alvarez E, Qian P, Wray S, et al. Ublituximab versus Teriflunomide in Relapsing Multiple Sclerosis. N Engl J Med. 2022;387(8):704-14.
26. Sun Y, Yang Y, Wang Z, Jiang F, Chen Z, Wang Z. Ozanimod for Treatment of Relapsing-Remitting Multiple Sclerosis in Adults: A Systematic Review and Meta-Analysis of Randomized Controlled Trials. Front Pharmacol. 2020;11:589146.
27. Kappos L, Radue EW, O'Connor P, Polman C, Hohlfeld R, Calabresi P, et al. A Placebo-Controlled Trial of Oral Fingolimod in Relapsing Multiple Sclerosis. N Engl J Med. 2010;362(5):387-401.
28. Cohen JA, Barkhof F, Comi G, Hartung HP, Khatri BO, Montalban X, et al. Oral Fingolimod or Intramuscular Interferon for Relapsing Multiple Sclerosis. N Engl J Med. 2010;362(5):402-15.
29. Jain N, Bhatti MT. Fingolimod-associated macular edema. Neurology. 2012;78(9):672-80.
30. Arvin AM, Wolinsky JS, Kappos L, Morris MI, Reder AT, Tornatore C, et al. Varicella-Zoster Virus Infections in Patients Treated With Fingolimod: Risk Assessment and Consensus Recommendations for Management. JAMA Neurol. 2015;72(1):31.
31. Thiel S, Langer-Gould A, Rockhoff M, Haghikia A, Queisser-Wahrendorf A, Gold R, et al. Interferon-beta exposure during first trimester is safe in women with multiple sclerosis—A prospective cohort study from the German Multiple Sclerosis and Pregnancy Registry. Mult Scler J. 2016;22(6):801-9.
32. Pauliat E, Onken M, Weber-Schoendorfer C, Rousson V, Addor MC, Baud D, et al. Pregnancy outcome following first-trimester exposure to fingolimod: A collaborative ENTIS study. Mult Scler J. 2021;27(3):475-8.
33. Comi G, Kappos L, Selmaj KW, Bar-Or A, Arnold DL, Steinman L, et al. Safety and efficacy of ozanimod versus interferon beta-1a in relapsing multiple sclerosis (SUNBEAM): a multicentre, randomised, minimum 12-month, phase 3 trial. Lancet Neurol. 2019;18(11):1009-20.
34. Cohen JA, Comi G, Arnold DL, Bar-Or A, Selmaj KW, Steinman L, et al. Efficacy and safety of ozanimod in multiple sclerosis: Dose-blinded extension of a randomized phase II study. Mult Scler J. 2019;25(9):1255-62.
35. Cree BA, Selmaj KW, Steinman L, Comi G, Bar-Or A, Arnold DL, et al. Long-term safety and efficacy of ozanimod in relapsing multiple sclerosis: Up to 5 years of follow-up in the DAYBREAK open-label extension trial. Mult Scler J. 2022;28(12):1944-62.
36. Kappos L, Fox RJ, Burcklen M, Freedman MS, Havrdová EK, Hennessy B, et al. Ponesimod Compared With Teriflunomide in Patients With Relapsing Multiple Sclerosis in the Active-Comparator Phase 3 OPTIMUM Study: A Randomized Clinical Trial. JAMA Neurol. 2021;78(5):558.
37. Kappos L, Li DKB, Stüve O, Hartung HP, Freedman MS, Hemmer B, et al. Safety and Efficacy of Siponimod (BAF312) in Patients With Relapsing-Remitting Multiple Sclerosis: Dose-Blinded, Randomized Extension of the Phase 2 BOLD Study. JAMA Neurol. 2016;73(9):1089-98.
38. Cao L, Li M, Yao L, Yan P, Wang X, Yang Z, et al. Siponimod for multiple sclerosis. Cochrane Database Syst Rev. 2021;11(11):CD013647.
39. Cohen JA, Coles AJ, Arnold DL, Confavreux C, Fox EJ, Hartung HP, et al. Alemtuzumab versus interferon beta 1a as first-line treatment for patients with relapsing-remitting multiple sclerosis: a randomised controlled phase 3 trial. Lancet. 2012;380(9856):1819-28.
40. Coles AJ, Twyman CL, Arnold DL, Cohen JA, Confavreux C, Fox EJ, et al. Alemtuzumab for patients with relapsing multiple sclerosis after disease-modifying therapy: a randomised controlled phase 3 trial. Lancet. 2012;380(9856):1829-39.
41. Ziemssen T, Bass AD, Berkovich R, Comi G, Eichau S, Hobart J, et al. Efficacy and Safety of Alemtuzumab Through 9 Years of Follow-up in Patients with Highly Active Disease: Post Hoc Analysis of CARE-MS I and II Patients in the TOPAZ Extension Study. CNS Drugs. 2020;34(9):973-88.
42. Giovannoni G, Comi G, Cook S, Rammohan K, Rieckmann P, Sørensen PS, et al. A Placebo-Controlled Trial of Oral Cladribine for Relapsing Multiple Sclerosis. N Engl J Med. 2010;362(5):416-26.
43. Sorensen PS, Pontieri L, Joensen H, Heick A, Rasmussen PV, Schäfer J, et al. Real-world experience of cladribine treatment in relapsing-remitting multiple sclerosis: A Danish nationwide study. Mult Scler Relat Disord. 2023;70:104491.

44. Krämer J, Bar-Or A, Turner TJ, Wiendl H. Bruton tyrosine kinase inhibitors for multiple sclerosis. Nat Rev Neurol. 2023;19(5):289-304.
45. Krupp L, Banwell B, Chitnis T, Deiva K, Gaertner J, Ghezzi A, et al. Effect of fingolimod on health-related quality of life in paediatric patients with multiple sclerosis: results from the phase 3 PARADIG MS Study. BMJ Neurol Open. 2022;4(1):e000215.
46. Chitnis T, Banwell B, Kappos L, Arnold DL, Gücüyener K, Deiva K, et al. Safety and efficacy of teriflunomide in paediatric multiple sclerosis (TERIKIDS): a multicentre, double-blind, phase 3, randomised, placebo-controlled trial. Lancet Neurol. 2021;20(12):1001-11.
47. Vermersch P, Scaramozza M, Levin S, Alroughani R, Deiva K, Pozzilli C, et al. Effect of Dimethyl Fumarate vs Interferon β-1a in Patients With Pediatric-Onset Multiple Sclerosis: The CONNECT Randomized Clinical Trial. JAMA Netw Open. 2022;5(9):e2230439.

CHAPTER 3

Progressive Forms of Multiple Sclerosis: Management

Subhas Bhuin, Areca Wangnoo, Padma Srivastava

ABSTRACT

Multiple sclerosis (MS) is a chronic disease with recurrent, subacute, focal neurologic symptoms, and signs that involves phases of diseases in which patients may improve or may evolve into a relentless progressive decline of neurologic functioning. Progressive phase of MS is the main determinant of onset of disability and its progression. Progressive MS patients have evidence of ongoing inflammation. Progression is not uniform over time and can include periods of relative stability or slow insidious change that is difficult to measure. Certain parameters predict a treatment response in progressive disease and analysis of those factors may aid in selection of patients responsive to and benefit from treatment to suppress inflammation and slow disability progression. This chapter enumerates the current and practiced treatment options with ongoing future trials and therapies in progressive MS. Along with approved drugs (ocrelizumab, siponimod, mitoxantrone, interferon, etc.), future therapy trials with *Bruton tyrosine kinase inhibitors such as evobrutinib and tolebrutinib* are included in the chapter. Measure of disability progression and treatment response is monitored with The Expanded Disability Status Scale (EDSS) score, Multiple Sclerosis Functional Composite (MSFC) consisting of timed 25-foot walk score (T25FW), 9-hole peg test score (9-HPT), and Paced Auditory Serial Addition Test (PASAT-3) with Symbol Digit Modalities Test (SDMT) and low-contrast assessment of visual acuity. Patient-reported outcomes measurements (PROMs) reflect the limitation of quality of life with higher likelihood of disability progression quantifiable patient feedback. Multidisciplinary team approach and rehabilitation support with palliative care to patient and caregiver support services are an important part of therapy in progressive MS patients with disability.

Keywords: Progressive phase of multiple sclerosis, The Expanded Disability Status Scale, Ocrelizumab, Bruton tyrosine kinase inhibitors.

INTRODUCTION

Multiple sclerosis (MS) is a chronic disease characterized by inflammation and demyelination of the central nervous system (CNS) associated with variable degrees of axonal and neuronal damage. It usually presents with recurrent, subacute, focal neurologic symptoms, and signs that may improve or may evolve into a relentless progressive decline of neurologic functioning.[1,2]

PHASES IN MULTIPLE SCLEROSIS[1,3-5]

- The *relapsing-remitting MS (RRMS)* is characterized by the presence of multiple clinically distinct events affecting different parts of the CNS separated in time (arbitrarily defined as at least 1 month apart) and subsequent improvement of neurological symptoms.
- *Progressive phase*: The progressive phase of MS is to be established after 1 year of clinical progression. During this phase, patients can continue to have active disease with symptomatic relapses or asymptomatic MRI activity. The patient is then further described as having active progressive or inactive progressive MS.

DEFINITIONS OF PROGRESSIVE PHASES (FIG. 1)

- *Progressive disease (primary or secondary)* (US NMSS—United States National Multiple Sclerosis Society):[4,6]
  - *Clinical*: Steadily increasing objectively documented neurological dysfunction/disability without unequivocal recovery (fluctuations and phases of stability may occur)
  - *Imaging (MRI)*: Increasing number and volume of T1-hypointense lesions, brain volume loss (BAL), and changes in magnetic transfer imaging and diffusion tensor imaging
- *Primary progressive MS (PPMS) (2017 McDonald criteria)*:[7]
  - 1 year of disability progression (retrospectively or prospectively determined) independent of clinical relapse *plus*
  - *Two of the following three:*
    - 1 or more T2-hyperintense lesions characteristic of MS in one or more of the following brain regions: Periventricular, cortical, juxtacortical, or infratentorial
    - 2 or more T2-hyperintense lesions in the MRI spinal cord
    - Presence of cerebrospinal fluid (CSF)-specific oligoclonal bands (OCBs)

    (No distinction made between symptomatic and asymptomatic MRI lesions)
- *Secondary progressive MS (SPMS) (Lorscheider et al. 2016)*:[8]
  - Worsening of EDSS score occurring in absence of relapse confirmed after 3 months
    - *Three-strata progression magnitude*:
      - Increase in EDSS by 1.5 points if the previous EDSS before conversion to SPMS was 0

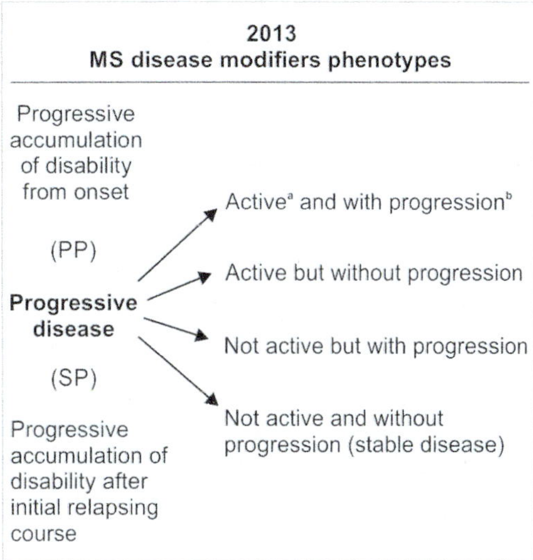

[a] *Activity* determined by clinical relapses and/or MRI activity (contrast-enhancing lesions, new or unequivocally enlarging T2 lesions) assessed at least annually

[b] *Progression*: Insidious and irreversible worsening of neurologic function due to MS over time (generally for more than 1 year), measured by clinical evaluation assessed at least annually

If assessments are not available, Activity and Progression are "indeterminate" MS.

FIG. 1: 2013 disease phenotype for both primary progressive (PP) multiple sclerosis (MS) and secondary progressive (SP) multiple sclerosis (MS).

Source: Adapted from Lublin FD, Reingold, SC, Cohen JA, Cutter GR, Sørensen PS, Thompson AJ, et al. Defining the clinical course of multiple sclerosis; 2013 revisions. Neurology. 2014;83(3):278-86.[6]

        - Increase in EDSS by 1 point if the previous EDSS was 1–5.5
        - Increase of EDSS by 0.5 points if the previous EDSS was >5.5
    - In the absence of a relapse, and
    - A minimum EDSS of ≥4
    - A pyramidal motor Functional Status (FS) score of ≥2
- SPMS is typically defined as deterioration independent of relapses for ≥6 months, following an initial RRMS course.[1,6]
- Patients with progressive clinical course >1 year but have single CNS demyelinating lesion, not fulfilling MS diagnosis criteria are considered having *progressive solitary sclerosis*[1]
- RRMS comprises 85% of all MS patients. If untreated around 85% of RRMS patients and if treated in disease-modifying therapy (DMT) era around 11.3% (in 10-year follow-up) patients of RRMS may develop secondary progression and gradual disability over time.[1,3]

MEASURES OF PROGRESSION IN PROGRESSIVE MULTIPLE SCLEROSIS[1,3,9-12]

Progression in PPMS and SPMS is not uniform over time and can include periods of relative stability or slow insidious change that is difficult to measure currently, multiple efforts are being made to identify and validate objective measures of progression.

- *The EDSS score* has been the main measure of clinical MS-related disability. Adding functional scores to the EDSS evaluation increases the ability to detect a reliable change over time.
- *MSFC* is a three-part, standardized, quantitative assessment instrument that integrates the following:
    - *Timed 25-foot walk (T25FW)* for leg function and ambulation
    - *9-HPT* for arm and hand function
    - *PASAT-3* for cognitive function was replaced eventually by the *SDMT, and low-contrast assessment of visual acuity* was added.[1,3,13-16]
- *PROMs*: They offer a structured way to quantify various symptoms such as fatigue, depression, and quality of life metrics, which were found to be worse in patients of progressive MS. In studies, evaluated parameters were Beck depression inventory-II (BDI-II), Multiple Sclerosis Impact Scale-29 (MSIS-29), and Fatigue Scale for Motor and Cognition (FSMC) in PPMS and SPMS. Worse performance in scores reflected the limitation of quality of life with higher likelihood of disability progression independent of relapse activity. They help in additional, practical, cost-efficient, and remotely accessible insight about disability progression in progressive MS patients through standardized, structured, and quantifiable patient feedback.[17]

FACTORS ASSOCIATED WITH THE DISEASE PROGRESSION[1,3,4,18-23]

- *Male gender*: Men especially older age at onset appear to exhibit shorter time to SPMS.
- *Age*:
    - Age has been long associated with progression in MS.
    - Older age is associated with reduced synaptic plasticity, less efficient remyelination, and impaired oligodendrocyte progenitors.
- *Race/ethnicity*: Studies identified African ancestry as a risk factor, not only for susceptibility to MS but also for disease progression and poorer disease outcomes.

- *Others*:
  - Type 2 diabetes, hypertension, and dyslipidemia
  - Tobacco and consumption
  - Obesity and low-serum 25-hydroxyvitamin D3 level
  - Vascular comorbidities and peripheral vascular disease
  - Spinal cord lesions
  - Slowed timed walk at baseline
  - Deterioration of EDSS score in first 2 years
  - Reduction in brain volume on MRI over 2 years
  - Increase in T2 lesion load and development of new lesions and cord atrophy over 2 years in MRI brain
  - Increasing gadolinium enhancing lesions in MRI brain
  - Absence of OCB in CSF associated with longer time to EDSS 6

RELAPSES IMPACT ON DISEASE PROGRESSION

- Fewer relapses in first 2–5 years of disease onset (early relapses) associated with longer time to disability and onset of progression in most studies.
- Later relapses (occurring >5–10 or >10 years after onset) had a minimal effect on long-term disease progression (either EDSS 6 or secondary progression).
- Relapses have greater impact on disease progression depending on age as a factor (< 25 years at MS onset has greater impact than older patients >35 years at MS onset).
- Complete or near complete recovery from first attack is indicative of slower progression to disability (secondary progression).
- Once SPMS and PPMS patients reach EDDS 4, and the rate of disability progression was same irrespective of relapses *(Confavreux and colleges study)*.[1,20,21]

MANAGEMENT OF PROGRESSIVE MULTIPLE SCLEROSIS

There are three drugs currently approved for progressive forms of MS (SPMS): Interferon beta (IFN-β), siponimod, and mitoxantrone. Ocrelizumab has been approved for the management of PPMS.

- The drugs aim to prevent inflammation by targeting either T or B cells. Many of the therapies tested carry risks (particularly infections), and thus it becomes important to select patients with progressive disease that will respond to these drugs so that benefit outweighs the risks associated with therapy.
- The studies use the definition of sustained disability progression as ≥1.0 point increase in patient's EDSS of up to 5.0 or 5.5 at baseline or ≥0.5 point increase in those with EDSS of >5.5, sustained for 3 months.
- Data indicate that in patients with PPMS, those who are younger and have more active disease will derive the greatest benefit from treatment.[6,24-32]

Interferon Therapy

- Many large randomized placebo controlled trials of IFN-β have shown a significant slowing of disease in SPMS and PPMS. Patients with a more rapid rate of EDSS progression seemed to benefit most from therapy (signs of ongoing inflammation may predict patients who may respond to this therapy).
- *SPECTRIMS (Secondary Progressive Efficacy Clinical Trial of Recombinant IFN*-β1a in MS) (Rebif 22 and 44 μg 3 times a week in SPMS) and *the IMPACT trial (International MS Secondary Progressive Avonex Controlled Trial) (Avonex 60 μg once a week in SPMS)* both did not show any effect on the time to confirmed

disease progression (CDP) as measured by EDSS but indicated significant effects on MRI parameters (Gd-enhancing and T2 lesions) and relapse rates for both the drugs.
- Statistical differences in MSFC score, T1 and T2 lesions volume and active lesions, and decrease in number of T2 lesions were seen with IFN-β1b compared to placebo.[1,4,5]

Mitoxantrone

- It is a cytotoxic DNA intercalating agent, which blocks topoisomerase II.
  Dosage is 12 mg/m^2 with 3 monthly dosages. It was approved by Food and Drug Administration (FDA) in 2000 for SPMS, progressive relapsing MS (PRMS), and worsening RRMS.
- A significant slowing of disability progression is measured by the EDSS, and ambulation index was observed in patients with RRMS and SPMS in MIMS trial (mitoxantrone in progressive MS), and other studies when treated with 12 mg/m^2 of mitoxantrone every 3 months with positive effects on the relapse rate and MRI parameters.
- Significant side effects included nausea, urinary tract infections, menstrual abnormalities, leukopenia, and decreased left ventricular ejection fraction, cardiotoxicity.
- Despite the positive outcome in patients with SPMS, negative results were reported in a smaller and shorter PPMS trial with mitoxantrone.[1,4,5,33]

Siponimod

- Sphingosine 1 phosphate antagonist (SIP) specifically blocks SIP1 and SIP5 receptors, hence preventing egression of lymphocytes from lymphoid tissues.
- It was approved by FDA for active SPMS in March 2019. The maintenance dose is 2 mg/day (except in CYP2C9 certain genotype is 1 mg/day). (*Testing for CYP29 genotype should be done before initiation due to dose medication requirement. Patients homozygous for CYP2C9*3/*3 should not receive the drug*)
- The EXPAND study and other studies in SPMS patients with siponimod had significant reduction to timed to 3-month confirmed disability progression (CDP) and 6-month CDP, but no benefit was seen in measures of worsening ambulatory dysfunction as measured by T25FW. Persons with relapses in the preceding 2 years or rapid progression had the most relative risk reduction.[4,34,35]
- The effect on disability progression was less pronounced in patients with increasing age, disability, disease duration, or less evidence of inflammatory disease. There was a trend toward a more favorable response in younger patients.
- A recent post hoc analysis assessed cognitive processing speed and found siponimod to have a clinically significant benefit in Symbols Digits Modality Test scores.
- *Second-generation sphingosine 1 receptor blockers (siponimod, ozanimod, ponesimod)* are approved for MS spectrum (clinically isolated syndrome to SPMS).[1,4,5]
- Adverse effects consist of heart failure, myocardial infarction or heart block, and macular edema with seizures are found to be more common as side effects.[1,4,5,35]

Ozanimod

- Selective S1P receptor 1 and 5 modulator (sphingosine 1 phosphate)
- Approved for use in adults with clinical isolated syndrome (CIS), RRMS, and active SPMS
- Dose is 0.92 mg once daily orally after initial day up titration.
- Trials showed decreased annualized relapse rate, new/enlarging T2 lesions, and decreased Gd-enhancing lesions.

- Contraindicated in patients taking monoamine oxidase inhibitor or with untreated severe sleep apnea[3]

Ponesimod

- An oral S1P receptor 1 modulator approved for use in CIS, RRMS, and active SPMS.
- Dosage of 2 mg oral once day with initial up titration.
- Randomized controlled trials showed decreased annualized relapse rate and decreased Gd-enhancing lesions by 58% by week 108 (from baseline).
- No statistical difference was seen in CDP between treatment groups.[3,5]

Ocrelizumab

- Humanized anti-CD20 monoclonal antibody is studied in the treatment for relapsing form of MS (including clinically isolated syndrome), active secondary progressive disease, and PPMS.
- Dose of initial 600 mg administered as two separate intravenous (IV) infusions over 2.5 hours, first as 300 mg IV followed by second 300 mg IV infusion. Subsequent doses are administered as single 600 mg IV infusion over 3.5–4 hours every 6 months.[1,3-5]
- *ORATORIO trial*: Patients received ocrelizumab 600 mg (administered as two 300 mg infusions given 2 weeks apart) or matching placebo every 24 weeks for a minimum of five doses (120 weeks)
  - Delay of clinical progression in patients with PPMS was seen with significant reduction in development to 12-week CDP and 24-week CDP. T25FW at week 120, T2W MRI lesions in brain and percentage of BAL were all found to be significantly reduced. Clinical benefits were maintained over ≥7.5 study years of treatment.
  - The high prevalence of inflammatory disease may have contributed to the positive outcome of the trial. A stronger consideration should be given to treat those younger and in early stages of PPMS.[4,36-40]
- *The ORATORIO-HAND study*:
  - It investigated the effects of ocrelizumab on upper limb function in patients with PPMS.
  - Ocrelizumab was found to be protective against the progression of upper extremity impairment, reducing the risk of 12-week or 24-week 9-HPT progression relative to placebo.[4,36,37]
- *Open-label extension phase study*:
  - The majority (97%) of the patients who completed the double-blind treatment period (to week 144) of ORATORIO entered the open-label extension (OLE) phase, during which all patients received ocrelizumab and followed for ≥ 6.5 study years (*one study year is equal to 48 weeks*).
  - They had lower rates of progression on most measures of 24-week CDP, which included EDSS progression rate, 9HPT completion time, T25FW. The benefits were found to be sustained over ≥6.5 years of treatment.
  - Lower rate of progression to requiring a wheelchair across the full study was found with delayed time to 24-week confirmed wheelchair requirement (i.e. EDSS ≥ 7.0) by 7.1 years relative to placebo.
  - In MRI outcomes, suppression of lesion activity was sustained (and near complete) over long-term treatment with ocrelizumab with lesser increases from baseline in T2 lesion volume and T1 hypointense lesion volume.[4,36-40]
- *Effectiveness of ocrelizumab in MS in a real-world clinical setting*:
  - Confirm the therapeutic benefits demonstrated in clinical trials.

 - CONFIDENCE study over one year of observation in PPMS and RRMS patients showed treatment success (defined as no relapse, no progression, or no treatment discontinuation due to an adverse event). Most patients were free of MRI disease activity after 1 year of treatment.
- The most common adverse effects were infusion-related reactions and infections such as herpes, varicella and respiratory tract infections. Hepatitis B virus screening is required before initiating therapy. Increased risk of malignancies is still uncertain.
- Meta-analyses generally indicate that ocrelizumab is superior or comparable to other approved DMTs in efficacy while being similar with respect to safety.
- With respect to patient convenience, ocrelizumab is infrequently administered (once every 6 months) and is minimally disruptive to the personal and professional lives of patients.[4,36,39]

Glatiramer Acetate

- The progressive MS trial in patients of PPMS showed no statistical difference in disease progression, but there was a decrease in number of new T2 bright lesions at year 2 and Gd-enhancing lesions in first year but not second year.
- There was a trend to lesser disability progression in men receiving glatiramer acetate compared to placebo, whereas men overall had a more rapid disability progression.[1,40]

Rituximab

- Chimeric antibody against CD20 with dosage of 500/1,000 mg IV 6 monthly. It was investigated in patients with PPMS.
- The primary outcome of time to CDP was negative, but significant effect on slowing of disability was seen in younger patients and in patients with at least 1 Gd-enhancing lesion at baseline. Although the accumulation of new T2 bright disease burden was lesser in rituximab patients at 2 years, no effect was found on brain volume.[1,3,41]

Cladribine

- It is a purine analog concentrated in lymphocytes and monocytes. It is approved for RRMS and active secondary progressive disease in patients with inadequate response to other drugs.
- Dose is 1.5 mg/kg/year taken as 10–20 mg/day for 4–5 days in a week 1 and 5. The dose is repeated 1 year later. No treatment is given in years 3 and 4.
- CLARITY trial and other studies of cladribine for progressive MS showed improvement on EDSS, Scripps Neurologic Rating scale, and MRI findings (decreased number and volume of Gd-enhancing lesions and decrease in accumulation of T2 bright lesions).
- Adverse effects included malignancy, teratogenicity, and acute heart failure with myocarditis with infection reactivations.[1,3,5,42,43]

Fingolimod

- The INFORMS study on fingolimod showed no significant difference between fingolimod and placebo groups in sustained improvement in EDSS.
- While it decreased the number of new/newly enlarging T2 lesions and the number of Gd+ T1 lesions on MRI relative to placebo, there was no significant difference between groups in BAL on MRI.
- In a separate study, fingolimod did slightly reduce microglial activation within focal lesions in microglial positron emission tomography (PET) imaging (reduction in PET signals), but not in the normal-appearing white matter.[3,4,44]

Intravenous Immunoglobulins

In PPMS and SPMS patients, placebo versus intravenous immunoglobulin (IVIg) at a dose of 0.4 mg/kg was infused for 24 months monthly. A small effect was seen on slowing of sustained disability progression in PPMS patients but not in SPMS patients. No MRI parameters were reported in this study.[1]

Natalizumab

- It is a monoclonal antibody against α1β4 integrin which was studied in SPMS trial (The ASCEND study) comprising EDSS, the T25FW test, and 9-HPT.
- No significant improvement was noted during 2 years of treatment, and no effect on EDSS progression and the T25FW test was seen.
- But an effect was seen on upper extremity function as measured by 9-HPT, suggesting performance measures may be more sensitive than EDSS for sustained worsening in progressive MS.[4,45]

Methotrexate

- Slowing of progression of upper limb in SPMS patients and PPMS patients were seen in patients who were administered low dose (7.5 mg) weekly methotrexate in study by Goodkin and colleagues.
- A decrease in new T2 lesions was seen correlating with lesser changes on the 9-HPT but not on the EDSS score.[1]

Cyclophosphamide

- It is an alkylating agent and broad suppressor of immune cells and cytokines.
- Dosage is induction (600 mg/m^2 IV plus IV methylprednisolone 1,000 mg/day for 5 days) followed by 700 mg/m^2 IV every other month for 2 years. A high-dose protocol (HiCy) with induction (50 mg/kg/day IV for 4 days) then 5 μg/kg/day IV granulocyte colony-stimulating factor.
- In patients of SPMS and PPMS with at least 1 point EDSS worsening during previous year, monthly pulses of cyclophosphamide showed 70% patients stabilized or improved on EDSS after 12 months of the treatment.
- Adverse effects include immunosuppression, hemorrhagic cystitis, hematological, and bladder carcinomas.[1,3,4]

Steroids

Intermittent steroids given by intrathecal injection in an open labeled trial showed no effect on the progression, whereas monthly IVMP in SPMS and PPMS patients with evidence of inflammation on MRI demonstrated a treatment effect.[1]

OTHER EMERGING THERAPIES[1,3,46-51]

- *High-dose biotin*: It is important in synthesis of myelin. 100 mg thrice daily for 12 months in a group of progressive MS patients study showed significant reversal of disability at 9 months (EDSS decrease of >1 point or >0.5 if EDSS 6 or 20% improvement in T25FW), which was confirmed at 12 months.
- *High-dose simvastatin*: Simvastatin trial in MS STAT 80 mg simvastatin versus placebo showed mean annualized atrophy rate lower in simvastatin group.
- *Lipoic acid*: It decreases the inflammation in optic and spinal cord. Medium effect on outcome was found in study of patients of SPMS patients who were assessed for timed up and go and quiet standing tasks using inertial sensors every 6 months for 2 years. Significant reduction in BVL was also found.
- *Ibudilast*: It is a phosphodiesterase inhibitor therapy inhibiting macrophage

migration. A double-blinded RCT trial (SPRINT MS) is being done. Studies showed slowing of progression of brain atrophy in PPMS patients.[47]

- *Opicinumab*: Antibody against LINGO 1 (inhibitor of oligodendrocyte differentiation axonal degeneration) has been investigated in a double-blinded trial (SYNERGY) in RRMS and SPMS patients which showed CDP improvement over 2 weeks.
- *Andrographolide*: An immunomodulator with neuroprotective properties has been investigated in patients of progressive MS who received 10 mg of oral drug twice daily for 24 months which showed significant difference in annualized mPBVC (mean percentage of brain volume change) on imaging.[1]

Future Therapies and Active Clinical Trials in Progressive Multiple Sclerosis

- *Riluzole, fluoxetine amiloride, N-acetyl cysteine, autologous stem cell transplantation, and pirfenidone are* involved in several open-label and cross-over studies which showed stabilization on various MRI and clinical outcomes.[1,44]
- *Bruton tyrosine kinase inhibitors*:[48,49]
    - CNS-penetrant BTK inhibitors might curtail disease progression by targeting CNS-compartmentalized B cells and microglia.
    - Currently five BTK inhibitors are being evaluated in progressive MS: *Evobrutinib, fenebrutinib, remibrutinib, tolebrutinib (all phase III trials), and orelabrutinib (phase II trial).*
    - In 24-week randomized double-blind trial, patients receiving 75 mg evobrutinib daily showed decreased Gd-enhancing lesions during 12–24 weeks. Though annual relapse rate and EDSS did not differ from placebo group. In OLE study, 75 mg twice daily was given, which showed reduction in annual relapse rate. It also showed reduction in neurofilament light chain levels maintained up to week 144.
    - Tolebrutinib 60 mg study showed decreased Gd-enhancing lesions, decreased annual relapse rates, and stable EDSS scores. Safety profile is still to be ascertained in chronic use.[46,48,49]
- *Vidofludimus calcium*: Inhibitor of dihydroorotate dehydrogenase (DHODH) oral available drug once a day which has shown a reduction of active and new MRI lesions is being studied in progressive and relapsing forms of MS.[46,50]
- *Foralumab*:
    - An investigational anti-CD3 agent (monoclonal antibody) which modulated T-cell function was studied in small-scale patients of nonactive SPMS, which showed improvements in clinical measures of fatigue and physical function.
    - Intranasal foralumab 50 µg/day 3 times a week for 2 weeks with 1 week rest, and assessment was done every 3 weeks.
    - Improvement in EDSS, T25FW test, pyramidal score, Modified Fatigue Impact Score (MFIS), and microglial PET imaging (reduction in PET signals) at 6 months was seen.
    - The therapy was shown to be safe with self-limited runny nose and nasal congestion as only treatment related adverse events. Further studies are being planned.[51]

CONTINUATION OR DISCONTINUATION OF DISEASE-MODIFYING THERAPY

- Trial is undergoing to examine effect of disease-modifying therapy discontinuation in patients older than 55 years and nonactive disease (which is defined as no evidence of recent new inflammatory disease with no relapse for at least 5 years and no new MRI lesion for at least 3 years).

- Recommendations have been suggested to stop therapy in those with SPMS who do not have ongoing relapses (or Gd-enhancing lesions on MRI activity) and have not been ambulatory (EDSS score 7 or greater) for at least 2 years.
- Older age, longer periods of stable disease on DMT with absent relapses or MRI activity, and an EDSS score less than 6 are associated with a low risk of disease worsening when stopping DMT use. In contrast, younger age (younger than 45 years) and a higher number of inflammatory lesions on MRI are predictive of resumption of disease activity.
- If discontinuation of DMT is decided, continued monitoring for breakthrough disease and rebound inflammatory activity is highly recommended.[3,5,52]

MULTIDISCIPLINARY CARE AND PALLIATIVE CARE IN PROGRESSIVE MULTIPLE SCLEROSIS

- Rehabilitation and symptom management are needed.
- Cognitive decline, falls, bladder, bowel impairments, pseudobulbar affect, fatigue, and mood changes worsen over time, which negatively affect quality of life. Other conditions mimicking progression should be identified including musculoskeletal conditions (knee and hip injuries) with comorbidities.
- Many patients with progressive disease who are restricted to home during the COVID-19 pandemic and have led to generalized worsening can be misclassified as progression.
- Weight control and stopping tobacco use, control of hypertension, hyperlipidemia, diabetes mellitus, and vascular disease are recommended.
- Encouragement to follow a healthy diet, exercise regularly and stretch, and maintain sleep hygiene is also recommended.
- Rehabilitation support should also include caregiver support services, tending to the emotional needs of both the patient and caregiver.[3,5,53-58]

CONCLUSION

- Common themes were found among all the progressive disease cohorts from the results of all evidence trials and other studies.
- Subset of patients with progressive MS may still have evidence of ongoing inflammation as evidenced as Gd-enhancing lesions, new T2 lesions (SPMS and PPMS), and relapses (SPMS).
- Certain parameters including gender might predict a treatment response in progressive disease due to subgroup of patients having faster disability progression making of detection of treatment effect easier.
- Inflammation and progressive tissue loss are integral components of all MS types. Multiple factors including genetic immunologic, environmental hormonal, and aging may interact to produce quantitative rather than qualitative differences, and further analysis of those factors that influence the clinical subtypes may aid in selection of patients responsive to treatment.
- It may therefore be possible to identify patients with progressive disease who may benefit from DMTs to suppress inflammation and slow disability progression.

- Careful selection may prevent exposure of patients to drugs with concerning risks without significant benefit. Thus, it may be feasible to identify patients with certain clinical and MRI characteristics whose progression is more rapid. Further evidence needs to be obtained on this aspect.[1]

REFERENCES

1. Srivastava Padma MV, PM Yogesh. Progressive forms of multiple sclerosis. Clinical Practice of Multiple Sclerosis and Related Disorders, 2nd edition. 2022. pp. 217-31.
2. Confavreux C, Composton A. The natural history of multiple sclerosis. In: Compston A (Ed). McAlpine's Multiple Sclerosis. London: Churchill Livingston: Elsevier; 2006. pp. 183-272.
3. Ontaneda D. Progressive Multiple Sclerosis. Continuum (Minneap Minn). 2019;25(3):736-52.
4. Pozzilli C, Pugliatti M, Nikolaos P, Grigoriadis N, Alkhawajah M, Airas L, et al. Diagnosis and treatment of progressive multiple sclerosis: A position paper. Eur J Neurol. 2023;30(1):9-21.
5. Amezcua L. Progressive Multiple Sclerosis. Continuum (Minneap Minn). 2022;28(4):1083-103.
6. Lublin FD, Reingold SC, Cohen JA, Cutter GR, Sørensen PS, Thompson AJ, et al. Defining the clinical course of multiple sclerosis: the 2013 revisions. Neurology. 2014;83(3):278-86.
7. Thompson AJ, Banwell BL, Barkhof F, Carroll WM, Coetzee T, Comi G, et al. Diagnosis of multiple sclerosis: 2017 revisions of the McDonald criteria. Lancet Neurol. 2018;17(2):162-73.
8. Lorscheider J, Buzzard K, Jokubaitis V, Spelman T, Havrdova E, Horakova D, et al. Defining secondary progressive multiple sclerosis. Brain. 2016;139(9):2395-405.
9. Lassmann H, van Horssen J, Mahad D. Progressive multiple sclerosis: pathology and pathogenesis. Nat Rev Neurol. 2012;8(1):647-56.
10. Kurtzke JF. Rating neurologic impairment in multiple sclerosis: an expanded disability status scale (EDSS). Neurology. 1983;33(11):1444-52.
11. Fischer JS, Rudick RA, Cutter GR, Reingold SC. The Multiple Sclerosis Functional Composite Measure (MSFC): an integrated approach to MS clinical outcome assessment. National MS Society Clinical Outcomes Assessment Task Force. Mult Scler. 1999;5(4):244-50.
12. Goldman MD, Motl RW, Scagnelli J, Pula JH, Sosnoff JJ, Cadavid D. Clinically meaningful performance benchmarks in MS: timed 25-foot walk and the real world. Neurology. 2013;81(21): 1856-63.
13. Orbach R, Zhao Z, Wang YC, O'Neill G, Cadavid D. Comparison of disease activity in SPMS and PPMS in the context of multicenter clinical trials. PLoS One. 2012;7(10):e45409.
14. Marrie RA. Comorbidity in multiple sclerosis: implications for patient care. Nat Rev Neurol. 2017;13(6):375-82.
15. Poser CM, Paty DW, Scheinberg L, McDonald WI, Davis FA, Ebers GC. New diagnostic criteria for multiple sclerosis: guidelines for research protocols. Ann Neurol. 1983;13(3):227-31.
16. Leray E, Yaouanq J, Le Page E, Coustans M, Laplaud D, Oger J, et al. Evidence for a two-stage disability progression in multiple sclerosis. Brain. 2011;133(7):1900-13.
17. Abdelhak A, Antweiler K, Kowarik MC, Senel M, Havla J, Zettl UK, et al. Patient-reported outcome parameters and disability worsening in progressive multiple sclerosis. Mult Scler Relat Disord. 2024;81:105-39.
18. Conway BL, Zeydan B, Uygunoğlu U, Novotna M, Siva A, Pittock SJ, et al. Age is a critical determinant in recovery from multiple sclerosis relapses. Mult Scler J. 2019;25(13):1754-63.
19. Paz Soldán MM, Novotna M, Abou Zeid N, Kale N, Tutuncu M, Crusan DJ, et al. Relapses and disability accumulation in progressive multiple sclerosis. Neurology. 2015;84(1):81-8.
20. Confavreux C, Vukusic S. Natural history of multiple sclerosis: a unifying concept. Brain. 2006;129:606-16.
21. Confavreux C, Vukusic S, Adeline P. Early clinical predictors and progression of irreversible disability in multiple sclerosis. Brain. 2003;126: 70-82.
22. Tutuncu M, Tang J, Zeid NA, Kale N, Crusan DJ, Atkinson EJ, et al. Onset of progressive phase is an age-dependent clinical milestone in multiple sclerosis. Mult Scler J. 2013;19(2):188-98.
23. Novotna M, Paz Soldán MM, Abou Zeid N, Kale N, Tutuncu M, Crusan DJ, et al. Poor early relapse recovery affects onset of progressive disease course in multiple sclerosis. Neurology. 2015;85(8):722-9.

24. Novotna M, Conway B, Zeydan B, Paz Soldan M, Abou Zeid N, Kale N, et al. Predicting the end of symptomatic relapses and disease modifying treatment use decisions in progressive multiple sclerosis [abstract S24.001]. Neurology. 2016;86(16 Suppl):S24-001.
25. Weideman AM, Tapia-Maltos MA, Johnson K, Greenwood M, Bielekova B. Meta-analysis of the age-dependent efficacy of multiple sclerosis treatments. Front Neurol. 2017;8:577.
26. Mackenzie I, Morant S, Bloomfield GA, MacDonald TM, O'Riordan JI. Changing face of multiple sclerosis in the United Kingdom 1990–2010. An incidence and prevalence study. J Neurol Neurosurg Psychiatry. 2013;84(11):e2.
27. Lassmann H, Horssen J, Mahad D. Progressive multiple sclerosis: pathology and pathogenesis. Nat Rev Neurol. 2012;8(11):647-56.
28. Baecher-Allan C, Kaskow BJ, Weiner HL. Multiple sclerosis: mechanisms and immunotherapy. Neuron. 2018;97(4):742-68.
29. Pitarokoili K, Gold R. Multiple sclerosis: progressive multifocal leukoencephalopathy risk stratification. Nat Rev Neurol. 2017;13(12):710-12.
30. Ontaneda D, Fox RJ, Chataway J. Clinical trials in progressive multiple sclerosis: lessons learned and future perspectives. Lancet Neurol. 2015;14(2):208-23.
31. Cross A, Riley C. Treatment of multiple sclerosis. Continuum (Minneap Minn). 2022;28(4):1025-51.
32. Hartung HP, Gonsette R, Konig N, Kwiecinski H, Guseo A, Morrissey SP, et al. Mitoxantrone in progressive multiple sclerosis: a placebo-controlled, double-blind, randomised, multicentre trial. Lancet. 2002;360(9350):2018-25.
33. Kappos L, Bar-Or A, Cree BAC, Fox RJ, Giovannoni G, Gold R, et al. Siponimod versus placebo in secondary progressive multiple sclerosis (EXPAND): a double-blind, randomised, phase 3 study. Lancet 2018;391(10127):1263-73.
34. Benedict RHB, Tomic D, Cree BA, Fox R, Giovannoni G, Bar-Or A, et al. Siponimod and cognition in secondary progressive multiple sclerosis: EXPAND secondary analyses. Neurology. 2021;96(3):e376-86.
35. Holloman JP, Axtell RC, Monson NL, Wu GF. The role of B cells in primary progressive multiple sclerosis. Front Neurol. 2021;12:680581.
36. Montalban X, Hauser SL, Kappos L, et al. Ocrelizumab versus placebo in primary progressive multiple sclerosis. N Engl J Med. 2017;376(3):209-20.
37. Montalban X, Matthews PM, Simpson A, Petrie JL, Sammon C, Ramagopalan S, et al. Real-world evaluation of ocrelizumab in multiple sclerosis: A systematic review. Ann Clin Transl Neurol. 2023;10(3):302-11.
38. Lamb YN. Ocrelizumab: A Review in Multiple Sclerosis. Drugs. 2022;82(3):323-34.
39. Wu X, Wang S, Xue T, Tan X, Li J, Chen Z, et al. Disease-modifying therapy in progressive multiple sclerosis: a systematic review and network meta-analysis of randomized controlled trials. Front Neurol. 2024;15:1295770.
40. Wolinsky JS, Narayana PA, O'Connor P, Coyle PK, Ford C, Johnson K, et al. Glatiramer acetate in primary progressive multiple sclerosis: results of a multinational, multicenter, double-blind, placebo-controlled trial. Ann Neurol. 2007;61(1):14-24.
41. Hawker K, O'Connor P, Freedman MS, Calabresi PA, Antel J, Simon J, et al. Rituximab in patients with primary progressive multiple sclerosis: results of a randomized double-blind placebo-controlled multicenter trial. Ann Neurol. 2009;66(4):460-71.
42. Giovannoni G, Comi G, Cook S, Rammohan K, Rieckmann P, Sørensen PS, et al. A placebo-controlled trial of oral cladribine for relapsing multiple sclerosis. N Engl J Med. 2010;362(5):416-26.
43. Rice GP, Filippi M, Comi G; Cladribine MRI Study Group. Cladribine and progressive MS: clinical and MRI outcomes of a multicenter controlled trial. Neurology. 2000;54(5):1145-55.
44. Lublin F, Miller DH, Freedman MS, Cree BA, Wolinsky JS, Weiner H, et al. Oral fingolimod in primary progressive multiple sclerosis (INFORMS): a phase 3, randomised, double-blind, placebo-controlled trial. Lancet. 2016;387(10023):1075-84.
45. Kapoor R, Ho PR, Campbell N, Chang I, Deykin A, Forrestal F, et al. Effect of natalizumab on disease progression in secondary progressive multiple sclerosis (ASCEND): a phase 3, randomised, double-blind, placebo-controlled trial with an open-label extension. Lancet Neurol. 2018;17(5):405-15.
46. Sriwastava S, Elkhooly M, Amatya S, Shrestha K, Kagzi Y, Bhatia D, et al. Recent advances in the treatment of primary and secondary progressive Multiple Sclerosis. J Neuroimmunol. 2024;390:578315.
47. Fox RF, Coffey CS, Conwit R, Cudkowicz ME, Gleason T, Goodman A, et al. Phase 2 trial of ibudilast in progressive multiple sclerosis. N Engl J Med. 2018;379(9):846-55.

48. Krämer J, Bar-Or A, Turner TJ, Wiendl H. Bruton tyrosine kinase inhibitors for multiple sclerosis. Nat Rev Neurol. 2023;19:289-304.
49. Airas L, Bermel RA, Chitnis T, Hartung HP, Nakahara J, Stuve O, et al. A review of Bruton tyrosine kinase inhibitors in multiple sclerosis. Ther Adv Neurol Disord. 2024;17:1-17.
50. Muehler A, Peelen E, Kohlhof H, Gröppel M, Vitt D. Vidofludimus calcium, a next generation DHODH inhibitor for the Treatment of relapsing-remitting multiple sclerosis. Mult Scler Relat Disord. 2020;43:102129.
51. Chitnis T, Kaskow BJ, Case J, Hanus K, Li Z, Varghese JF, et al. Nasal administration of anti-CD3 monoclonal antibody modulates effector CD8+ T cell function and induces a regulatory response in T cells in human subjects. Front Immunol. 2022;13:956907.
52. Kaminsky AL, Omorou AY, Soudant M, Pittion-Vouyovitch S, Michaud M, Anxionnat R, et al. Discontinuation of disease-modifying treatments for multiple sclerosis in patients aged over 50 with disease inactivity. J Neurol. 2020;267(12):3518-27.
53. Clare L, Teale JC, Toms G, Kudlicka A, Evans I, Abrahams S, et al. Cognitive rehabilitation, self-management, psychotherapeutic and caregiver support interventions in progressive neurodegenerative conditions: a scoping review. NeuroRehabilitation. 2018;43(4):443-71.
54. Spain R. Approach to symptom management of multiple sclerosis with a focus on wellness. Continuum (Minneap Minn). 2022;28(4):1052-82.
55. Wachterman MW, Pilver C, Smith D, Ersek M, Lipsitz SR, Keating NL. Quality of end-of-life care provided to patients with different serious illnesses. JAMA Intern Med. 2016;176(8):1095-102.
56. Lee YJ, Yoo JW, Hua L, Kim PC, Kim SJ, Shen JJ. Ten-year trends of palliative care utilization associated with multiple sclerosis patients in the United States from 2005 to 2014. J Clin Neurosci. 2018;58:13-9.
57. Oliver DJ, Borasio GD, Caraceni A, De Visser M, Grisold W, Lorenzl S, et al. A consensus review on the development of palliative care for patients with chronic and progressive neurological disease. Eur J Neurol. 2016;23(1):30-8.
58. Solari A, Giordano A, Sastre-Garriga J, Köpke S, Rahn AC, Kleiter I, et al. EAN guideline on palliative care of people with severe, progressive multiple sclerosis. J Palliat Med. 2020;23(11):1426-43.

CHAPTER 4

Switching Therapies in Multiple Sclerosis

Kamakshi Dhamija, Sitla Prasad Pathak

ABSTRACT

With increasing advancements in the field of multiple sclerosis (MS) therapeutics, switching among various disease-modifying therapies is a common clinical challenge. Treatment failures and drug intolerance remain the most prevalent reasons for switching. Apart from these, various drug and patient-related factors can influence decision-making. Moreover, no universal guidelines exist for definition of threshold for a switch in therapy, given the diversity of clinical situations which can arise in day-to-day practice. We aim to discuss various factors and tools that can guide clinical decisions for therapy switching in MS.

Keywords: Multiple sclerosis, Disease modifying therapy, Treatment switch, Treatment failure.

INTRODUCTION

Multiple sclerosis (MS) is an autoimmune demyelinating condition of the central nervous system, which predominantly affects younger age population, especially females. As the number of disease-modifying therapies (DMTs) increase, the treatment decisions for initiation, switching, and deescalating the treatment also become increasingly complex. Once a diagnosis of MS is made, further discussion centers on valid treatment options for a particular patient keeping in mind the relative efficacy of DMTs, cost concerns, feasibility of monitoring, potential short- and long-term side effects, concerns pertaining to pregnancy and childbirth, among other factors. Likewise, when deciding on switching therapies, similar factors come into play. This chapter focuses on various factors involved in switching DMTs and aims to provide a framework for management decisions.

POTENTIAL REASONS FOR SWITCHING THERAPIES

The decision to switch therapies in people with MS (PwMS) can be patient or physician driven.[1] There may be drug-centered factors such as cost of the drug, its availability, tolerance, side effects, and efficacy. Some patient-driven factors might influence the decision of switching to another drug, of which the most important one remains the aggressiveness of the disease and occurrence of relapses despite being on a DMT. There may be adherence issues, or in other scenarios, pregnancy and childbirth can influence the switch decisions. Sometimes, the physician's familiarity with the administration of the drug might also influence treatment decisions. With the current availability of a host of treatment options for MS, it is logically possible to tailor a DMT for a particular patient. However, no universal guideline can encompass all scenarios which the physicians face in day-to-day practice. Among reasons for switching DMTs, perhaps the leading ones remain lack of treatment efficacy and adverse effects. The key questions pertaining to decisions on switching DMTs include the following:

When do We Consider Treatment Failure in Case of Multiple Sclerosis Therapies?

In clinical practice, two treatment regimens are often debated in MS: The escalation regimen and early highly efficacious therapy (HET) approach. With the tremendous advent of high-efficacy drugs, the concept of "*hit early hit hard*" has gathered its roots in MS therapeutics. The current practice trends widely include the initiation of higher-efficacy drugs at the outset, especially when the disease is highly active and switching down to medium-efficacy drugs after a period of disease control (flipping the pyramid).[2] **Table 1** depicts the categorization of MS drugs according to their efficacy. Clearly, patients who fail the first DMT require timely switching to a second higher-efficacy DMT. There is wide heterogeneity with the concept of treatment response and nonresponse and the consideration of time frame for defining failure of treatment in MS. Complicating assessment is that DMTs take time to work. Broadly, three outcomes which are assessed in evaluation of the treatment response are incurrence of fresh relapses, progression of disability, and appearance of inflammatory activity on magnetic resonance imaging (MRI) (new T2/flair lesions or contrast-enhancing lesions).[3]

Indicators of Clinical Response—the Relapses

Relapses are the hallmark of relapsing remitting MS (RRMS) and prevention of relapses is one of the most targeted goals in MS trials, as well as one of the key parameters of no evidence of disease activity (NEDA). If a patient relapses while on a DMT, some key facts to consider before switching therapies in MS include the timing since a patient has been on a particular DMT, compliance to therapy, the severity and "recovery" from relapse, and

TABLE 1: Categorization of drugs for MS.[4-6]

Efficacy category	Drugs
Low–moderate efficacy DMTs	Interferons
	Glatiramer acetate
	Teriflunomide
Moderate efficacious	Fumarates as dimethyl fumarate, diroximel fumarate
Moderate to highly efficacious	Sphingosine 1 receptor modulators as fingolimod, siponimod, ponesimod, and ozanimod
	Cladribine
Highly effective therapies	Natalizumab
	B-cell depleters—ocrelizumab, rituximab, ofatumumab
	Alemtuzumab

(DMTs: disease-modifying therapies; MS: multiple sclerosis)

a reasonable exclusion of "pseudorelapse." It should be noted that DMTs take time to work. This "therapeutic lag" was assessed in a study including data from two MS registries: MSBase (multinational) and OFSEP (French). For 10 therapies assessed, therapeutic lag ranged from 12 to 30 weeks [mean of 12.7 weeks for fingolimod and 30.2 weeks for dimethyl fumarate (DMF)].[7] The delay to treatment effect was even longer when disability progression was considered ranging from 30 to 70 weeks for seven therapies in the same study. Higher disability scores, annualized relapse rates ≥ 1, and male gender were associated with longer therapeutic delays for disability progression.[8] Hence, after due consideration of the drug-related pharmacodynamic factors, an early decision to switch to a higher-efficacy medication should be taken in case of a relapse.

Indicators of Treatment Response—the Disability Progression

Relapses and progression are two important clinical indicators of disability in MS. The natural history of MS has shown that once the disability in MS becomes clinically evident, it is no longer determined by the presence of previous relapses. Hence, disability progression might be a more important clinical surrogate than the occurrence of relapses in MS.[9] Disability in MS has two aspects: Relapse-associated worsening (RAW) in RRMS and progression independent of relapse activity (PIRA) in progressive MS forms. PIRA, the silent progression in MS, has been reported to occur at the rate of 2–5% per year and can occur in those patients who remain in NEDA-3 in the first treatment years.[10] Hence, the assessment of disability progression is vital for consideration of switch in therapies. Typically, a 1.0-point increase in expanded disability status scale (EDSS) at 6 months after initiating a DMT is considered as disability progression resulting from treatment failure.[11] This endpoint has been extrapolated from studies with short-to-medium follow-up. In studies with long-term follow-up over 15–16 years, a net increase in EDSS,[12] transition to secondary progressive MS (SPMS), and attaining EDSS of ≥6 is also considered as disability progression.[13] Disability progression on first DMT mandates escalation of treatment. Nevertheless, we must understand that activation of innate immune system is linked to disability progression in MS. Early initiation of highly effective therapy in MS might reboot the immune system and pave way in halting the mechanisms responsible for disability progression in MS. This advocates for early HET initiation, rather than waiting for the progression to happen and losing the opportunity to treat.

Indicators of Treatment Response—the Disease Activity on MRI

Disease activity on MRI is assessed by new T2/flair lesions, enlarging T2 lesions, or the presence of gadolinium-enhancing lesions on follow-up MRI. Increasing T2 lesion volume, emergence of new T2 lesions, and inflammatory activity on MRI in initial 1–2 years of therapy initiation have been identified as poor prognostic factors for disability progression in interferon-treated patients.[14,15] The "lesion threshold" for a therapy switch has been variably considered in literature, and differential importance has been given to contrast-enhancing lesions as well.[11,16] However, MRI assessment of lesions has got few technical limitations. Three-dimensional (3D)-Flair is the core sequence for diagnosis and monitoring in MS radiology.[17] In the absence of availability of these highly sensitive sequences, assessment is usually done on the available T2/flair sequences, which tends to have inter-individual variability. This might have a good reliability for contrast-enhancing lesions, lesser though for new or enlarging T2 lesions.[18] MRI-acquisition protocols vary from center to center, especially the contrast administration strategy, timing of acquiring the image after contrast administration, and the contrast dose. It is important to be aware of these external factors before considering treatment failure.

Another concept of importance is the rebaselining of MRI after initiation of a DMT. DMTs have a therapeutic lag and if a change in therapy is considered based on a pre-DMT scan, there are chances that the drug might not have received its share of effect to cast a radiological change. A "rebaselining MRI" should be done 3–6 months after a therapy switch.[14] Treatment effectiveness, without clinical relapses, should be determined with further annual MRIs. Gadolinium-enhanced scans are not recommended for usual follow-up studies; however, they may add predictive value in the rebaseline scan.[17] One important lack in our current practice is the failure to realize that the T1 black holes are also an important marker of axonal loss and neuronal destruction; hence, accumulating T1 black hole burden is a marker of therapy failure, although we lack sufficient evidence to support a therapy switch in this setting.[19]

Defining Treatment Failure

According to the European consensus publications, definite treatment failures are those patients with ≥3 new T2 lesions and 1 relapse or ≥2 relapses, independent of MRI activity in 6–12 months despite DMT. American guidelines are stricter and consider treatment failure for patients with ≥1 relapse or ≥2 new MRI lesions. Clearly enlarged T2 lesions also count as new MRI lesions.[3] With respect to the disability, treatment failure is considered as a 1-point increase in EDSS confirmed at 1-year follow-up.[20] Patients with treatment failures are candidates for intensification of DMTs (vertical switch) **(Fig. 1)**.

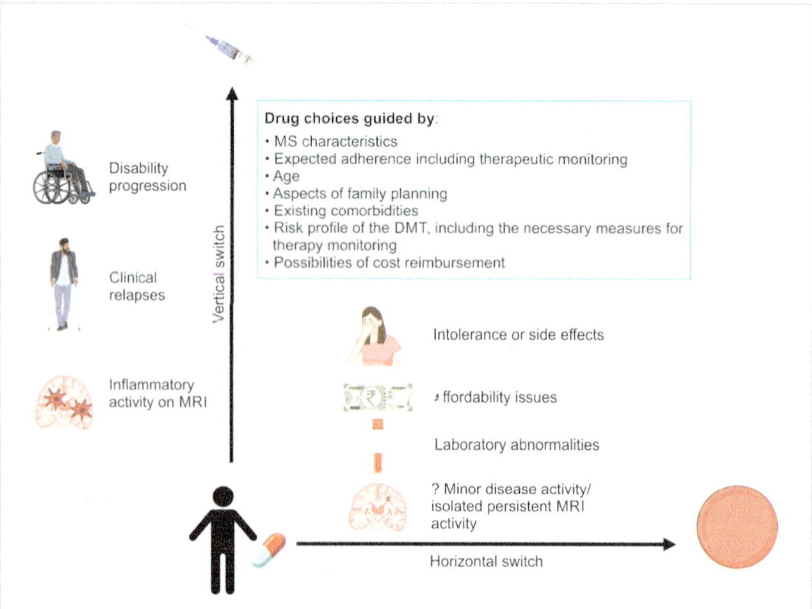

FIG. 1: Types of switches in MS therapeutics.

(DMT: disease-modifying therapy; MRI: magnetic resonance imaging; MS: multiple sclerosis)

What should be the Treatment Goals for Switching Therapies?

With the advent of highly effective therapies in MS, the concept of *NEDA* has emerged as a potential therapeutic goal. NEDA-3 is a composite of three clinical and radiological measures of disease activity, i.e., (1) no relapses, (2) no disability progression, and (3) no MRI activity (new or enlarging T2 lesions or gadolinium-enhancing lesions).[21] The concept of NEDA-3 is based predominantly on recognition of "neuroinflammatory" component of the disease rather than the "neurodegenerative" part. With more stringent treatment goals and increasing thrive to target the degenerative aspect of the disease, there is increasing inclusion of other parameters in NEDA definition as brain atrophy (brain volume loss <0.4% per year; NEDA-4) and certain other parameters as cognition and biomarkers as well (definitions yet to be elucidated).[4,21] However, for all practical purposes, NEDA-3 remains the most assessable goal in real-world settings. While NEDA is a "zero-tolerance" concept, some recent studies have aimed to define a level of disease activity while on DMT which can be tolerated without disability worsening. This concept of minimal evidence of disease activity (MEDA) corresponds to having no clinical relapse and ≤2 new focal T2 lesions in absence of contrast-enhancing lesions.[22] The MEDA concept is based on MRI in MS (MAGNIMS) low stratification risk and is discussed in subsequent sections. Nevertheless, for all practical purposes, unless clearly attributable to treatment nonadherence, many MS neurologists are prompted for treatment escalation with any new asymptomatic MRI activity while on platform DMTs. In rare situations, minor radiological activity (e.g., <2 lesions on follow-up scan) or isolated persistent radiological activity might prompt for a horizontal switch of DMTs.

Are there Any Objective Scores Available for Guiding a Therapy Switch?

Few of the subsequently described scoring systems can be useful in guiding management decisions for switching therapies. However, it must be borne in mind that it is difficult for any predefined clinicoradiological criteria to encompass all the clinical scenarios encountered in everyday practice and the scoring systems remain useful "guiding tools" at their best.

Rio Score[16]

Rio et al. developed a logistic model for evaluation of disease activity in patients on platform therapy (interferon-beta).[16] The score was developed with an intent to identify early nonresponders as treatment changes after a long period of observation (2–3 years) might not remain meaningfully effective for the patients. Rio score is calculated by adding one point each for (1) at least one relapse, (2) at least three new MRI lesions, and (3) a sustained deterioration in EDSS score by ≥1 point over a period of 1 year. Patients with at least two of these three variables analyzed after 12 months of treatment were seen to have a high risk for clinical activity and disease progression after 3 years, hence for escalation of treatment [odds ratio (OR) 5.9–13.2]. Over subsequent 8 years of follow-up, Rio score ≥ 2 at 1 year had an accuracy of 77% in predicting EDSS worsening over this time.[23]

Modified Rio Score[24]

The modified Rio score was developed by Sormani and coworkers after the work of Rio et al. This score is based on only new T2 lesions and relapses, since combination of these two factors accounts for almost 100% of treatment effect on disability worsening at 2 years. The modified Rio score-stratified patients into three risk groups according to the probability of disability worsening, utilizing a cutoff of four or more lesions on MRI and the occurrence of relapses. The risk score categories include: Low (score 0), intermediate (score 1), and high risk (score 2–3) after 1 year of therapy with interferon beta-1a. This had an excellent specificity (97%) and very low sensitivity (24%) in discriminating treatment response. The modified Rio score was further refined to include a new clinical visit and a repeat brain MRI at 6 months after the first treatment year in order to allow a better risk stratification of patients in the medium risk group, who were most difficult to classify in terms of future treatment response.[25]

MAGNIMS Score[26]

In a large clinical dataset collected by the MAGNIMS (MRI in MS) network, three risk categories have been proposed. The scoring system utilizes the number of relapses and new T2 lesions after first year of platform DMT use (interferon-beta). Low-risk (score 0) group is defined as no relapses and minimal focal MRI activity (0–2 new T2 lesions). This group was found to have a negligible probability of disability worsening in the following 2–3 years. Medium-risk group was defined as either no relapses and ≥3 new T2 lesions or 1 relapse and 0–2 new T2 lesions. This group requires an additional clinical and MRI follow-up (i.e., rebaseline) after the first year of treatment to overcome uncertainty about treatment effect. High-risk group is defined as more than two clinical relapses or one relapse and three T2 lesions. The risk of failure in this group is around 48%.[26]

To ease the concerns, the Canadian MS working group released the recommendations for modification of therapy, which included not only the components of NEDA but a space for the severity of relapses as well.[27] The same is illustrated in **Table 2.**

What Therapies should be Switched to in Case of Treatment Failures?

Switch in therapies can be either a horizontal switch from platform therapies (as interferon and glatiramer acetate) to DMF or teriflunomide or a vertical switch to HET. Robust evidence now supports that in case of treatment failures, horizontal switch results in a higher relapse rate and a trend toward less EDSS improvement than vertical switching.[28] HET also has a significant effect on lowering the risk of RAW and PIRA.[29] Previous studies have confirmed a definite advantage of "immediate" switching to HET rather than "delayed" switching.[3] **Table 3** illustrates key

TABLE 2: Recommendations for switching therapies in MS.[27]

	Minor	Major
Relapse rate	One relapse in first 2 years of treatment	>2 relapses in first 2 years of treatment
Severity	• Mild • No functional impairment • No motor/cerebellar/brainstem/ sphincter involvement	• Moderate to severe • Functional impairment • Motor/cerebellar/brainstem/sphincter involvement
Recovery	• Full recovery at 6 months • No functional impairment • EDSS change by <1 point at 6 months	• Incomplete recovery • Functional impairment • EDSS change by >1 point at 6 months
MRI	One new lesion	>3 new lesions during treatment

Note: An escalation in treatment is warranted if patient meets any of the major criteria.

(EDSS: expanded disability status scale; MRI: magnetic resonance imaging)

TABLE 3: Summary of studies pertaining to switch in therapies for MS.

Authors	Study details	Summary of key findings
Carrá et al., 2008[32]	Therapeutic outcome 3 years after switching of immunomodulatory therapies in patients with relapsing remitting multiple sclerosis in Argentina	Patients were switched either from low-dose to high-dose IFN-β ($n = 31$), from IFN-β to GA ($n = 52$) or mitoxantrone ($n = 13$), or from GA to IFN-β ($n = 16$). Least improvement was observed in patients switching between INF-β preparations. Median EDSS scores remained stable in all groups except the GA to IFN-β switchers. Patients who fail first-line immunomodulatory therapy generally benefit from switching to another class of immunomodulatory therapy
Castillo-Trivino et al., 2011[33]	Switching multiple sclerosis patients with breakthrough disease to second-line therapy	Relapse rate decreased by 70% in switchers to natalizumab and by 77% in switchers to immunosuppressants. Insignificant relapse rate reduction was seen among nonswitchers ($p = 0.87$). Switching to natalizumab or immunosuppressants in patients with breakthrough disease activity was significantly effective
Coles et al., 2012[34]	Alemtuzumab for patients with relapsing multiple sclerosis after DMT: a randomized controlled phase 3 trial	Adults with at least one relapse on IFN-β or glatiramer were randomly allocated in 1:2:2 ratio to receive IFN-β-1a 44 μg, alemtuzumab 12 mg or alemtuzumab 24 mg (discontinued later on). 51% patients in the IFN-β-1a group relapsed compared with 35% of patients in the alemtuzumab group ($p < 0.0001$), corresponding to a 49.4% improvement with alemtuzumab
Prosperini et al., 2012[35]	Escalation to natalizumab or switching among immunomodulators in relapsing MS	An escalation to natalizumab is more effective than switching among immunomodulators in RRMS patients who failed a first-line treatment
Bergvall et al., 2014[36]	Relapse rates in patients with MS switching from interferon to fingolimod or glatiramer acetate: A US claims database study	Patients with MS who switched from interferons to fingolimod were significantly less likely to experience relapses than those who switched to glatiramer
Fox et al., 2014[37]	Outcomes of switching directly to oral fingolimod from injectable therapies: Results of the randomized, open-label, multicenter, EPOC study in relapsing MS	Treatment satisfaction improved significantly in patients who switched to fingolimod compared with those who continued injectable DMT. Patients also reported significant improvements in health-related quality of life, reduced depression, and reduced fatigue severity after a switch to fingolimod
He et al., 2015[38]	Comparison of switch to fingolimod or IFN-β/glatiramer acetate in active MS	Patients had received fingolimod, interferon-beta, or glatiramer acetate for a minimum of 3 months following a switch of immunomodulatory therapy were included in the study. Switching from injectable immunomodulators to fingolimod is associated with fewer relapses, more favorable disability outcomes, and greater treatment persistence compared with switching to another injectable preparation following on-treatment activity of MS

Continued

Continued

Authors	Study details	Summary of key findings
Spelman et al., 2015[39]	Comparative efficacy of switching to natalizumab in active MS	Compared to switching between IFN-β and GA, switching to natalizumab reduced annualized relapse rate in year one by 65–75%, the risk of first relapse by 53–82% (mean follow-up 1.7–2.2 years) and treatment discontinuation events by 48–65% (all $p \leq 0.001$)
Braune et al., 2016[40]	Efficacy of fingolimod is superior to injectable DMT in second-line therapy of relapsing remitting MS	Fingolimod showed statistically significant superior efficacy in comparison to injectable DMT regarding annualized relapse rate (0.21 vs. 0.33 per year), time-to-relapse and likelihood of relapse (injectable DMT HR 1.7), proportion and likelihood of patients with EDSS progression (15.10% vs. 31.00%; injectable DMT HR 1.7), persistence on medication and likelihood of discontinuation (injectable DMT HR 3.0). Significantly more patients were free of relapse and EDSS progression with fingolimod than with their second injectable DMT (64.4% vs. 46.5%; $p < 0.03$)
Vermersch et al., 2022[41]	Efficacy and safety of ocrelizumab in patients with RRMS with suboptimal response to prior DMT: A primary analysis from the phase 3b CASTING single-arm, open-label trial	In patients switching therapy due to suboptimal disease control, treatment with ocrelizumab led to an overall high NEDA rate across a wide range of disease-related and demographic subgroups, regardless of prior treatment background, with no new safety signals detected
Guger et al., 2023[28]	Effects of horizontal versus vertical switching of disease-modifying treatment after platform drugs on disease activity in patients with RRMS in Austria	Horizontal switching after a platform therapy resulted in a higher relapse and interrupt probability and was associated with a trend toward less EDSS improvement compared to vertical switching in Austrian RRMS patients
Marriott et al., 2023[42]	Switching to second-line MS DMTs is associated with decreased relapse rate	Switching to second-line DMTs was associated with a longer time to treat relapse in comparison to those who remained on a first-line DMT (HR 0.44; 95% CI 0.32–0.62, $p < 0.0001$). Thus, switching to high-efficacy DMTs reduces the rates of subsequent MS relapse at the population level

(CI: confidence interval; DMT: disease-modifying therapy; EDSS: expanded disability status scale; EPOC: Evaluate Patient OutComes; GA: glatiramer acetate; HR: hazard ratio; IFN-β: interferon-beta; MS: multiple sclerosis; NEDA: no evidence of disease activity; RRMS: relapsing remitting MS)

trials' results for switching of DMTs in MS. With all this evidence, Multiple Sclerosis Therapy Consensus Group (MSTCG) guidelines recommend immediate shifting to HET in the case of clinicoradiological activity with mild-to-moderately efficacious DMTs.[3] Various other guidelines as EAN/ECTRIMS also recommend the same.[30] A few studies have also tried to address other factors associated with therapy switching. Younger age, diagnostic delay, higher EDSS scores, and spinal cord lesions were independently found to be associated with higher switch rates.[31] Unanimously, the evidence remains strong for switching to HET in case of treatment failures.

What are the Recommendations for Switching in Case of Drug-related Side Effects?

There are frequent clinical scenarios wherein DMTs require switching if a patient develops intolerance to ongoing treatment. In the setting of intolerance to therapy with adverse effects or complications, lateral switch to equipotent DMTs may be reasonable. Comorbidities were found to be associated with more probability of lateral switching.[31] Persistent laboratory abnormalities such as leukopenia or transaminitis may also be a factor for lateral switching.[43] Concerns for side effects also remain a call for switching DMTs, especially John Cunningham virus (JCV) serostatus.

Categorization of Progressive Multifocal Leukoencephalopathy Risk

Disease-modifying therapies have been stratified into three categories according to progressive multifocal leukoencephalopathy (PML) risk.[44] Of this, the only drug with class I risk for PML is natalizumab. Class II drugs with low but real risk of PML include DMF and fingolimod. Class III agents with very low or no risk of PML include alemtuzumab, ocrelizumab, and ofatumumab. Rituximab is also a class III agent; however, the risk of PML with this drug has been found to be 1 in 25,000 in patients with rheumatoid arthritis.[45] Till date, one patient with MS on rituximab developed PML; however, he had switched from natalizumab and developed PML within 6 months of the therapy switch.[46] Clinicians should discuss the risk of PML with patients on DMTs such as natalizumab, fingolimod, and DMF and consider switching if the patients turn JCV serostatus positive, especially if the titers are >0.9.[43] Patients on natalizumab who develop infusion reactions with the drug or who develop breakthrough disease activity should be checked for antibodies against the drug and if found persistently positive, they should also undergo a switch in therapy.[43] In a case of switching from natalizumab to another HET, risk of carryover PML should always be borne in mind and a MRI scan should be performed in view of same. In high suspects, cerebrospinal fluid (CSF) for JCV polymerase chain reaction (PCR) may guide decision-making.[3]

Should there be a Washout Period before Switching to Next Therapy?

The period of switching is crucial for the patients and has two important aspects to it. A shorter switch time exposes the patients to higher side effects, especially the infection risk. On the other hand, a longer switch time predisposes for rebound disease activity. Rebound disease activity can be severe in MS and can be seen as early as after 6 weeks of natalizumab discontinuation and 3 months of sphingosine-1 phosphate (S1P) receptor modulator drugs. Based on the French Multiple Sclerosis Society recommendations, washout period has been defined for various DMTs in use. **Table 4** illustrates recommended washout periods for therapy switch. For drugs that regularly

TABLE 4: Recommended washout periods for therapy switch.[47]

Drug	Washout period
Interferons	None
Glatiramer acetate	None
Teriflunomide	None
Dimethyl fumarate	None (especially in lymphocyte counts are >800/mm^3)
Fingolimod	1 month
Natalizumab	1 month
Ocrelizumab	3 months
Mitoxantrone	6 months

lead to lymphopenias, such as alemtuzumab, cladribine, or S1P receptor modulators, the lymphopenia should have largely regressed before switching if the patient's clinical condition permits a pause in therapy. The benefit-risk ratio should be assessed on case-to-case basis.[3]

CONCLUSION

Although we acknowledge that an earliest hint of persisting disease activity prompts the clinicians for therapy switch to highly effective drugs, the evidence strongly advocates the early initiation of HET in order to avoid disability in MS patients. Various objective scoring systems exist for categorization of this failure risk and can guide clinical decision-making. The therapies should always be tailored according to the disease and patient's characteristics. The essence of treatment optimization is the early recognition of treatment failure and prompt initiation of HET, saving the vital treatment responsive years in young MS population.

BEST PRACTICE PEARLS FOR SWITCHING THERAPIES IN MULTIPLE SCLEROSIS

- Hitting early means hitting hard in MS. Timely initiation of highly effective therapies in MS prevents disability progression.
- Clinicians should monitor the disease clinically, making an objective assessment of disability at each visit and performing at least annual MRIs to assess disease activity.
- There is a therapeutic lag in the initiation of treatment effect of DMTs and this should be considered before deciding to switch a therapy, especially if breakthrough activity is experienced early on.
- Although the threshold for treatment switching has been variably opined in literature, clinicians should discuss the switch decisions if a patient suffers one or more relapses, develops two or more unequivocally new MRI lesions, or experiences a decline in EDSS after 1 year of DMT use.
- Adherence to DMTs should always be ensured before decision for switching therapy.
- Intolerance to therapy might prompt a therapy switch to another equipotent DMT (horizontal switch). Intolerance to one DMT is a risk factor for inadherence to subsequent DMT also. Sometimes, minor disease activity may prompt a horizontal switch.
- In case of treatment failure, timely and immediate shift to highly effective therapies should be done (vertical switch).
- Knowledge about washout periods for DMTs can guide practical decision-making.

REFERENCES

1. Gross RH, Corboy JR. Monitoring, Switching, and Stopping Multiple Sclerosis Disease-Modifying Therapies. Contin Minneap Minn. 2019;25:715-35.
2. Giovannoni G. Multiple sclerosis should be treated using a step-down strategy rather than a step-up strategy-YES. Mult Scler J. 2016;22:1397-400.
3. Wiendl H, Gold R, Berger T, Derfuss T, Linker R, Mäurer M, et al. Multiple Sclerosis Therapy Consensus Group (MSTCG): position statement on disease-modifying therapies for multiple sclerosis (white paper). Ther Adv Neurol Disord. 2021;14:17562864211039648.
4. Roos I, Leray E, Frascoli F, Casey R, Brown JWL, Horakova D, et al. Delay from treatment start to full effect of immunotherapies for multiple sclerosis. Brain. 2020;143:2742-56.

5. Roos I, Leray E, Frascoli F, Casey R, Brown JWL, Horakova D, et al. Determinants of therapeutic lag in multiple sclerosis. Mult Scler. 2021;27:1838-51.
6. Casanova B, Quintanilla-Bordás C, Gascón F. Escalation vs. Early Intense Therapy in Multiple Sclerosis. J Pers Med. 2022;12:119.
7. Prosperini L, Ruggieri S, Haggiag S, Tortorella C, Pozzilli C, Gasperini C. Prognostic Accuracy of NEDA-3 in Long-term Outcomes of Multiple Sclerosis. Neurol Neuroimmunol Neuroinflamm. 2021;8:e1059.
8. Gasperini C, Prosperini L, Tintoré M, Sormani MP, Filippi M, Rio J, et al. Unraveling treatment response in multiple sclerosis. Neurology. 2019;92:180-92.
9. Bermel RA, You X, Foulds P, Hyde R, Simon JH, Fisher E, et al. Predictors of long-term outcome in multiple sclerosis patients treated with interferon β. Ann Neurol. 2013;73:95-103.
10. Goodin DS, Traboulsee A, Knappertz V, Reder AT, Li D, Langdon D, et al. Relationship between early clinical characteristics and long term disability outcomes: 16 year cohort study (follow-up) of the pivotal interferon β-1b trial in multiple sclerosis. J Neurol Neurosurg Psychiatry. 2012;83:282-7.
11. Hoffmann O, Gold R, Meuth SG, Linker RA, Skripuletz T, Wiendl H, et al. Prognostic relevance of MRI in early relapsing multiple sclerosis: ready to guide treatment decision making? Ther Adv Neurol Disord. 2024;17:17562864241229325.
12. Prosperini L, Gallo V, Petsas N, Borriello G, Pozzilli C. One-year MRI scan predicts clinical response to interferon beta in multiple sclerosis. Eur J Neurol. 2009;16:1202-9.
13. Rio J, Castilló J, Rovira A, Tintoré M, Sastre-Garriga J, Horga A, et al. Measures in the first year of therapy predict the response to interferon β in MS. Mult Scler J. 2009;15:848-53.
14. Wattjes MP, Ciccarelli O, Reich DS, Banwell B, de Stefano N, Enzinger C, et al. 2021 MAGNIMS-CMSC-NAIMS consensus recommendations on the use of MRI in patients with multiple sclerosis. Lancet Neurol. 2021;20:653-70.
15. Erbayat Altay E, Fisher E, Jones SE, Hara-Cleaver C, Lee JC, Rudick RA. Reliability of classifying multiple sclerosis disease activity using magnetic resonance imaging in a multiple sclerosis clinic. JAMA Neurol. 2013;70:338-44.
16. Sahraian MA, Radue E-W, Haller S, Kappos L. Black holes in multiple sclerosis: definition, evolution, and clinical correlations. Acta Neurol Scand. 2010;122:1-8.
17. Río J, Nos C, Tintoré M, Téllez N, Galán I, Pelayo R, et al. Defining the response to interferon-beta in relapsing-remitting multiple sclerosis patients. Ann Neurol. 2006;59:344-52.
18. Giovannoni G, Turner B, Gnanapavan S, Offiah C, Schmierer K, Marta M. Is it time to target no evident disease activity (NEDA) in multiple sclerosis? Mult Scler Relat Disord. 2015;4:329-33.
19. Newsome SD, Binns C, Kaunzner UW, Morgan S, Halper J. No Evidence of Disease Activity (NEDA) as a Clinical Assessment Tool for Multiple Sclerosis: Clinician and Patient Perspectives [Narrative Review]. Neurol Ther. 2023;12:1909-35.
20. Prosperini L, Mancinelli C, Haggiag S, Cordioli C, De Giglio L, De Rossi N, et al. Minimal evidence of disease activity (MEDA) in relapsing-remitting multiple sclerosis. J Neurol Neurosurg Psychiatry. 2020;91:271-7.
21. Río J, Rovira À, Tintoré M, Otero-Romero S, Comabella M, Vidal-Jordana Á, et al. Disability progression markers over 6-12 years in interferon-β-treated multiple sclerosis patients. Mult Scler. 2018;24:322-30.
22. Sormani MP, Rio J, Tintorè M, Signori A, Li D, Cornelisse P, et al. Scoring treatment response in patients with relapsing multiple sclerosis. Mult Scler. 2013;19:605-12.
23. Sormani M, Signori A, Stromillo M, De Stefano N. Refining response to treatment as defined by the Modified Rio Score. Mult Scler. 2013;19:1246-7.
24. Sormani MP, Gasperini C, Romeo M, Rio J, Calabrese M, Cocco E, et al. Assessing response to interferon-β in a multicenter dataset of patients with MS. Neurology. 2016;87:134-40.
25. Freedman MS, Devonshire V, Duquette P, Giacomini PS, Giuliani F, Levin MC, et al. Treatment Optimization in Multiple Sclerosis: Canadian MS Working Group Recommendations. Can J Neurol Sci. 2020;47:437-55.
26. Guger M, Enzinger C, Leutmezer F, Di Pauli F, Kraus J, Kalcher S, et al. Effects of horizontal versus vertical switching of disease-modifying treatment after platform drugs on disease activity in patients with relapsing–remitting multiple sclerosis in Austria. J Neurol. 2023;270:3103-11.
27. Kappos L, Wolinsky JS, Giovannoni G, Arnold DL, Wang Q, Bernasconi C, et al. Contribution of Relapse-Independent Progression vs. Relapse-Associated Worsening to Overall Confirmed Disability Accumulation in Typical Relapsing Multiple Sclerosis in a Pooled Analysis of 2 Randomized Clinical Trials. JAMA Neurol. 2020;77:1132-40.

28. Montalban X, Gold R, Thompson AJ, Otero-Romero S, Amato MP, Chandraratna D, et al. ECTRIMS/EAN guideline on the pharmacological treatment of people with multiple sclerosis. Eur J Neurol. 2018;25:215-37.
29. Saccà F, Lanzillo R, Signori A, Maniscalco GT, Signoriello E, Lo Fermo S, et al. Determinants of therapy switch in multiple sclerosis treatment-naïve patients: A real-life study. Mult Scler. 2019;25:1263-72.
30. Rae-Grant A, Day GS, Marrie RA, Rabinstein A, Cree BAC, Gronseth GS, et al. Practice guideline recommendations summary: Disease-modifying therapies for adults with multiple sclerosis. Neurology. 2018;90:777-88.
31. Berger JR. Classifying PML risk with disease modifying therapies. Mult Scler Relat Disord. 2017;12:59-63.
32. Clifford DB, Ances B, Costello C, Rosen-Schmidt S, Andersson M, Parks D, et al. Rituximab-Associated Progressive Multifocal Leukoencephalopathy in Rheumatoid Arthritis. Arch Neurol. 2011;68: 1156-64.
33. Luna G, Alping P, Burman J, Fink K, Fogdell-Hahn A, Gunnarsson M, et al. Infection Risks Among Patients With Multiple Sclerosis Treated With Fingolimod, Natalizumab, Rituximab, and Injectable Therapies. JAMA Neurol. 2020;77(2): 184-91.
34. Freeman L, Longbrake EE, Coyle PK, Hendin B, Vollmer T. High-Efficacy Therapies for Treatment-Naïve Individuals with Relapsing–Remitting Multiple Sclerosis. CNS Drugs. 2022;36:1285-99.
35. Lee C-Y, Chan K-H. Personalized Use of Disease-Modifying Therapies in Multiple Sclerosis. Pharmaceutics. 2024;16:120.
36. Carrá A, Onaha P, Luetic G, Burgos M, Crespo E, Deri N, et al. Therapeutic outcome 3 years after switching of immunomodulatory therapies in patients with relapsing–remitting multiple sclerosis in Argentina. Eur J Neurol. 2008;15:386-93.
37. Castillo-Trivino T, Mowry EM, Gajofatto A, Chabas D, Crabtree-Hartman E, Cree BA, et al. Switching Multiple Sclerosis Patients with Breakthrough Disease to Second-Line Therapy. PLoS One. 2011; 6:e16664.
38. Coles AJ, Twyman CL, Arnold DL, Cohen JA, Confavreux C, Fox EJ, et al. Alemtuzumab for patients with relapsing multiple sclerosis after disease-modifying therapy: a randomised controlled phase 3 trial. Lancet. 2012;380:1829-39.
39. Prosperini L, Giannì C, Leonardi L, De Giglio L, Borriello G, Galgani S, et al. Escalation to natalizumab or switching among immunomodulators in relapsing multiple sclerosis. Mult Scler. 2012;18:64-71.
40. Bergvall N, Makin C, Lahoz R, Agashivala N, Pradhan A, Capkun G, et al. Relapse Rates in Patients with Multiple Sclerosis Switching from Interferon to Fingolimod or Glatiramer Acetate: A US Claims Database Study. PLoS One. 2014;9:e88472.
41. Fox E, Edwards K, Burch G, Wynn DR, LaGanke C, Crayton H, et al. Outcomes of switching directly to oral fingolimod from injectable therapies: Results of the randomized, open-label, multicenter, Evaluate Patient OutComes (EPOC) study in relapsing multiple sclerosis. Mult Scler Relat Disord. 2014;3:607-19.
42. He A, Spelman T, Jokubaitis V, Havrdova E, Horakova D, Trojano M, et al. Comparison of Switch to Fingolimod or Interferon Beta/Glatiramer Acetate in Active Multiple Sclerosis. JAMA Neurol. 2015;72:405-13.
43. Spelman T, Kalincik T, Zhang A, Pellegrini F, Wiendl H, Kappos L, et al. Comparative efficacy of switching to natalizumab in active multiple sclerosis. Ann Clin Transl Neurol. 2015;2:373-87.
44. Braune S, Lang M, Bergmann A; NeuroTransData Study Group. Efficacy of fingolimod is superior to injectable disease modifying therapies in second-line therapy of relapsing remitting multiple sclerosis. J Neurol. 2016;263:327-33.
45. Vermersch P, Oreja-Guevara C, Siva A, Van Wijmeersch B, Wiendl H, Wuerfel J, et al. Efficacy and safety of ocrelizumab in patients with relapsing-remitting multiple sclerosis with suboptimal response to prior disease-modifying therapies: A primary analysis from the phase 3b CASTING single-arm, open-label trial. Eur J Neurol. 2022;29:790-801.
46. Marriott JJ, Ekuma O, Fransoo R, Marrie RA. Switching to second line MS disease-modifying therapies is associated with decreased relapse rate. Front Neurol. 2023;14:1243589.
47. Bigaut K, Cohen M, Durand-Dubief F, Maillart E, Planque E, Zephir H, et al. How to switch disease-modifying treatments in multiple sclerosis: Guidelines from the French Multiple Sclerosis Society (SFSEP). Mult Scler Relat Disord. 2021;53:103076.

CHAPTER 5

Management of NMOSD and MOGAD

Ayush Agarwal, Rohit Bhatia

ABSTRACT

Neuromyelitis optica spectrum disorder (NMOSD) and myelin oligodendrocyte glycoprotein antibody-associated disease (MOGAD) are antibody-mediated demyelinating disorders of the central nervous system (CNS). The main goals of management include treatment of an acute relapse and long-term immunomodulatory therapy for disease stability. Acute treatment involves use of steroids, plasmapheresis, IVIG alone or in combination. Although conventional immunosuppressive agents are still the most prescribed, newer agents have been approved for NMOSD. Treatment of MOGAD follows conventional immunosuppressive therapy. The present chapter outlines the therapeutic strategies for management of NMOSD and MOGAD.

Keywords: Neuromyelitis optica spectrum disorder (NMOSD), Myelin oligodendrocyte glycoprotein antibody-associated disease (MOGAD), Aquaporin-4 (AQP4), Relapse, Myelin oligodendrocyte glycoprotein immunoglobulin G (MOG-IgG), Myelin oligodendrocyte glycoprotein (MOG).

INTRODUCTION

Neuromyelitis optica spectrum disorder (NMOSD) and myelin oligodendrocyte glycoprotein antibody-associated disease (MOGAD) are antibody-mediated demyelinating disorders of the central nervous system (CNS).[1,2] Both have distinct biomarkers, antibodies against aquaporin-4 (AQP4) water channels on the astrocytes for NMOSD[3] and antibodies against myelin oligodendrocyte glycoprotein (MOG) for MOGAD.[4] The clinical overlap of these two disorders prevented their recognition for a long time as separate entities and they were initially considered as variants of multiple sclerosis (MS). Despite afflicting similar CNS regions (optic nerves and spinal cord), recent studies have highlighted the significant pathogenic and prognostic differences between NMOSD and MOGAD.[5]

Unlike MS, the disability in NMOSD and MOGAD is accrued only with repeated attacks/relapses, and disease progression in the absence of relapses has not been proven. There is no curative therapy for both and treatment entails two main goals: Treatment of an acute attack and prevention of future attacks.[6] The disease continues to relapse in the absence of the latter leading to significant disability. Unlike NMOSD and MS, approximately 50% of patients have a monophasic illness.[7,8] Recently, randomized controlled trials (RCTs) have led to the Food and Drug Administration's (FDA's) approval of multiple immunotherapies for adult patients with AQP4 antibody-positive NMOSD for relapse prevention. The diagnostic criteria of MOGAD were laid down by the International MOGAD panel in 2023[2] and multiple RCTs are ongoing to test the efficacy of monoclonal antibodies such as rituximab and satralizumab in MOGAD. The present chapter outlines the long-term preventive therapies for NMOSD and MOGAD.

NEUROMYELITIS OPTICA SPECTRUM DISORDER

Basics of Neuromyelitis Optica Spectrum Disorder Management

Anti-AQP4 antibodies are pathogenic in NMOSD and are present in approximately 80% NMOSD patients.[9] Antigen antibody reaction-associated inflammation is further enhanced by complement-mediated damage and associated cytotoxicity.[10,11] This finally leads to loss of astrocytic AQP4 expression (especially at the blood-brain barrier) resulting in astrocytic damage with increased permeability of the blood-brain barrier and secondary affliction of neurons and oligodendrocytes. Treatment includes immunosuppression—nonspecific (oral glucocorticoids, azathioprine, and mycophenolate mofetil) and specific targeted therapies [anti-CD20—rituximab, anti-CD19—inebilizumab, anti-interleukin 6 (IL-6)—satralizumab and tocilizumab, anti-complement—eculizumab].[12] A broad outline of NMOSD management is shown in **Flowchart 1**.

Treatment of Acute Attack

The detailed management of acute relapses is covered in another chapter. The neuromyelitis optica study group (NEMOS) revised recommendations advise that therapy should be initiated as early as possible with high-dose glucocorticoid therapy with or without plasmapheresis, depending upon the response.[6] The latter can be used as first line if history of insufficient response to

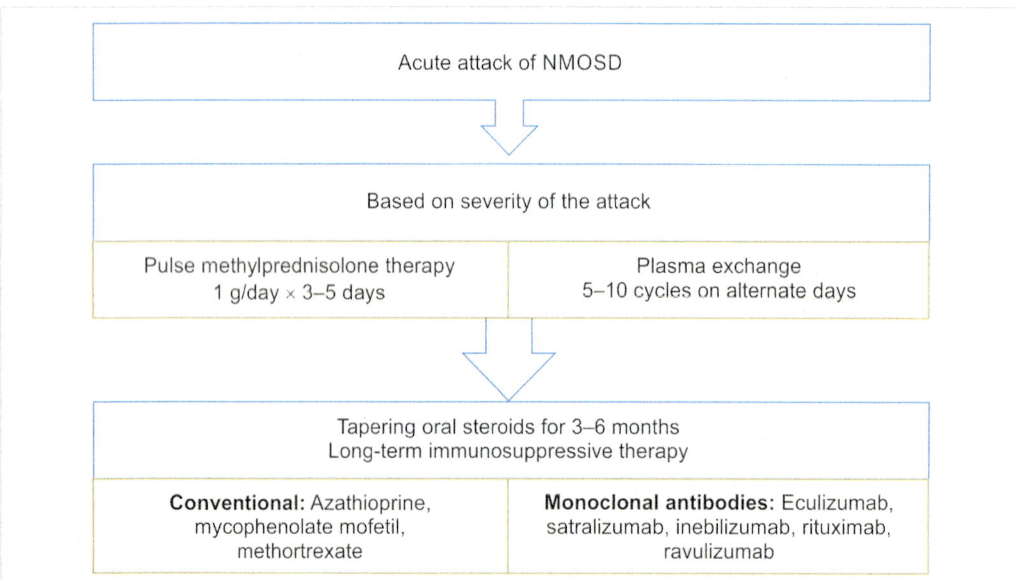

FLOWCHART 1: Management of neuromyelitis optica spectrum disorder (NMOSD).

glucocorticoids or good response to plasma exchange is present in previous attacks or severe presentations such as acute myelitis.[6]

Relapse Prevention

One of the key goals of NMOSD treatment is to prevent further relapses.[6] Unlike MS, there is no disease progression in the absence of attacks, and seropositive NMOSD invariably takes a relapsing course, with highest risk in the first few years.[13] Each attack can lead to permanent disability[14] and long-term immunosuppression should be started for patients with seropositive NMOSD after their first attack.[6] Previously, recommendations for long-term immunosuppression included treatment with azathioprine, mycophenolate mofetil, or rituximab and were based on retrospective data from case series and open-label trials. However, multiple RCTs in recent times on monoclonal antibodies have led to the FDA approval for four drugs for use in adult seropositive NMOSD—eculizumab, inebilizumab, satralizumab, and ravulizumab. **Table 1** outlines the commonly used agents in long-term disease control.

Conventional Immunosuppressants

Oral Glucocorticoids

Glucocorticoids suppress the immune system through multiple mechanisms by binding to glucocorticoid receptors on lymphocytes (genomic and nongenomic). Prednisolone is the most commonly used oral steroid. Although these can be used in low doses for prolonged periods as the sole immunosuppressant, their use commonly leads to adverse effects such as weight gain, cushingoid habitus, hypertension, osteoporosis, and dyslipidemia. As a result, steroids are usually used as a bridging therapy, while other conventional immunosuppressants such as azathioprine and mycophenolate mofetil take effect. There is no data from RCTs on what the ideal dosing is, timing of tapering, or rate of steroid tapering. However, as a principle, steroids are usually started at a dose of 1 mg/kg and slowly tapered over time with a close watch on disease activity.

Azathioprine

Azathioprine is a widely available, affordable, effective treatment for NMOSD.[15] It is a purine analog which inhibits the activation and differentiation of lymphocytes.[15] Due to a lag of 4–6 months in its onset of action, it is usually combined with low-dose glucocorticoids for that duration.[16] Details on its dosing and side effects are mentioned in **Table 1**. Periodic blood counts and liver function monitoring are mandatory during azathioprine use.

Mycophenolate Mofetil

Mycophenolate mofetil is a prodrug that gets converted into mycophenolic acid and suppresses lymphocyte proliferation through inhibition of enzyme inosine-5'-monophosphate dehydrogenase, which leads to depletion of guanine nucleotides of B- and T-cells. It has a lag of 2–3 months in action onset, leading to the requirement of steroid bridging, like azathioprine.[17] Details on its dosing and side effects are mentioned in **Table 1**. Periodic blood counts and liver function monitoring are mandatory during mycophenolate mofetil use.

Monoclonal Antibodies

Eculizumab

Eculizumab is a humanized monoclonal antibody which is a terminal complement inhibitor. It prevents the association of C5 convertase with C5, preventing its cleavage into proinflammatory components C5a and C5b and thereby the terminal complement cascade.[18] Before its use in NMOSD, it was used for managing paroxysmal nocturnal hemoglobinuria, myasthenia gravis, and atypical hemolytic uremic syndrome. The potent complement-mediated neurotoxicity of the AQP4 antibody in NMOSD is likely offset by the complement inhibition of eculizumab, leading to efficacy. The

TABLE 1: Immunosuppressants used in the treatment of neuromyelitis optica spectrum disorder (NMOSD).

Drug	Clinical trial	Mechanism of action	Dosage	Side effects
Eculizumab	PREVENT[19]	Anti-C5 complement monoclonal antibody	Intravenous 900 mg/week × 4 doses 1,200 mg/fortnight thereafter	Meningococcal infection, URTI, headache, infusion reaction
Satralizumab	SAkuraStar SAkuraSky[22,23]	Anti-IL-6 monoclonal antibody	Subcutaneous 120 mg stat and weeks 2 and 4, 120 mg/month thereafter	Arthralgia, headache, infections
Inebilizumab	N-Momentum[25]	Anti-CD-19 monoclonal antibody	Intravenous 300 mg stat and week 2, 300 mg/6 monthly thereafter	Infections, infusion reaction
Azathioprine	–	Purine synthase inhibitor	Oral 2–3 mg/kg body weight	Leukopenia, anemia, deranged LFT, infections, malignancy
Mycophenolate mofetil	–	Inosine-5′-monophosphate dehydrogenase inhibitor	Oral 1–2 g/day	Leukopenia, anemia, deranged LFT, gastrointestinal symptoms
Tocilizumab	TANGO[24]	Anti-IL-6 monoclonal antibody	Intravenous infusion: 8 mg/kg/month	Arthralgia, headache, infections

(IL-6: interleukin 6; LFT: liver function test; N-MOmentum: Inebilizumab for the Treatment of Neuromyelitis Optica Spectrum Disorder; SAkuraSky: Trial of Satralizumab in Neuromyelitis Optica Spectrum Disorder; PREVENT: Eculizumab in Aquaporin 4-Positive Neuromyelitis Optica Spectrum Disorder; SAkuraStar: Safety and Efficacy of Satralizumab Monotherapy in Neuromyelitis Optica Spectrum Disorder; TANGO: Safety and Efficacy of Tocilizumab Versus Azathioprine in Highly Relapsing Neuromyelitis Optica Spectrum Disorder; URTI: upper respiratory tract infection)

PREVENT trial[19] was a multicenter, randomized, double-blind study comparing eculizumab to placebo, in seropositive adult-onset NMOSD conducted on AQP4-positive adult patients who had at least two attacks in the previous 6 months. It was observed that the proportion of patients who remained attack free was significantly greater in the eculizumab group compared to placebo at 1, 2, and 4 years of treatment. This treatment effect was independent of gender, ethnicity, and geographical location.[20] The effect of concomitant usage of immunosuppressive medications in the PREVENT trial[19] is of concern as approximately 70% of patients were receiving them. Another uncertainty is whether these results can be extrapolated to seronegative NMOSD patients and their safety in pregnancy. Eculizumab has a prompt onset of action and provides near-complete C5 activity inhibition after the first infusion.[6] It is recommended at a dose of 900 mg once a week for four doses followed by 1,200 mg once every fortnight.[18] Data on long-term safety of eculizumab is mainly extrapolated from use in other indications. Infections with encapsulated bacteria are a special concern and all patients should be vaccinated against *Neisseria* infections at least 4 weeks prior to starting eculizumab therapy.[6]

Ravulizumab

Ravulizumab is a newer-generation C5 complement inhibitor with similar efficacy[21] as eculizumab but with a major advantage of longer dosing intervals (once every 8 weeks) due to a longer half-life.

Satralizumab

Satralizumab is a humanized monoclonal antibody (immunoglobulin G2) which is an IL-6 receptor blocker and has been approved for use for both monotherapy and combination therapy in adult seropositive NMOSD patients. Satralizumab binds to both soluble and membrane-bound IL-6 receptors, thereby preventing IL-6 from binding to its receptor, hence reducing IL-6-mediated B- and T-cell activation. This inhibition prevents B-cell differentiation into AQP4-secreting plasma cells.

SAkuraStar and SAkuraSky were two multicentric, phase 3 randomized trials comparing satralizumab to placebo and satralizumab add-on to baseline immunotherapy to baseline immunotherapy alone, respectively. Both trials found a significant reduction in relapse rates with satralizumab.[22,23] Unlike eculizumab, no increased risk of infections with capsulated organisms was found and no deaths or anaphylactic reactions were reported in either trial. However, both the SAkuraStar and SAkuraSky trials did not show a statistically significant reduction in relapses in patients with seronegative NMOSD. Therefore, there is insufficient evidence for use in this patient population. Safety in pregnancy is also not established. It has a subcutaneous route of administration and is available in a 120 mg prefilled syringe. The recommended dose is 120 mg once every month.

Tocilizumab

Tocilizumab is an anti-IL-6 drug which has been used off-label in NMOSD and has been observed to be safe and effective. When compared to azathioprine, it significantly reduced the relapse risk in the open-label, multicentric, randomized, phase 2 TANGO trial.[24]

Inebilizumab

Inebilizumab is a humanized monoclonal antibody that targets CD19-positive B-cells and depletes them, including the pro-B stage (benefit over rituximab).[25-27] This is important since AQP4 is secreted throughout the B-cell life cycle including the pro-B stage. N-MOmentum was a multicentric, randomized, double-blind phase 2/3 trial which evaluated the safety and efficacy of inebilizumab. It found a statistically significant reduction in the number of relapses, magnetic resonance imaging (MRI) lesions, worsening of disability, and duration of hospital stay in patients who received inebilizumab.[25-27] The study also revealed decreased levels (12.9%) of serum glial fibrillary acidic protein (GFAP) (a marker of disease activity) in the inebilizumab arm.[25,28] Unlike eculizumab, no increased risk of infections with capsulated organisms was found and no deaths or anaphylactic reactions were reported. The rates of infusion reactions, arthralgias, and infections were also similar in both groups.[26,27] It is given as an intravenous infusion of 300 mg, 2 weeks apart, followed by 300 mg once every 6 months.[25]

MYELIN OLIGODENDROCYTE GLYCOPROTEIN ANTIBODY-ASSOCIATED DISEASE

Basics of Myelin Oligodendrocyte Glycoprotein Antibody-associated Disease Management

As in NMOSD, MOG-immunoglobulin G (IgG) antibodies are pathogenic, leading to antigen-antibody reactions and associated damage to the nervous system (oligodendrocytes and neurons). The production of antibodies and entry into CNS are facilitated by high levels of secreting IL-6.[29] Unlike NMOSD, intrathecal production of MOG antibodies has been reported.[30] Also, complement activation and associated neuronal damage is lesser in MOGAD as compared to NMOSD.[31] A broad outline of MOGAD management is shown in **Flowchart 2**.

Treatment of Acute Attack

The acute treatment of MOGAD attacks is similar to NMOSD. A recent study has also shown the utility of intravenous immunoglobulin (IVIg) in acute attacks of MOGAD attacks.[32] The detailed management of acute relapses is covered in another chapter.

Relapse Prevention

The approach to long-term immunosuppression may differ from NMOSD. There is a lack of consensus on the long-term immunosuppression after the first acute attack as approximately 50% of attacks of MOGAD may be monophasic.[2] Long-term follow-up data does suggest relapsing nature of the disease. Factors such as adult-onset disease, severe attack at presentation, incomplete recovery, and cord relapse may direct the decision to treat. This should be individualized after a clear explanation to the patient and an appropriate decision taken. We prefer to treat with prophylactic immunosuppression after the first attack.

None of the FDA-approved therapies for NMOSD have been tested in RCTs for MOGAD and are therefore used off-label on a common principle as we treat NMOSD or other autoimmune conditions.

Oral immunosuppressants such as azathioprine and mycophenolate have the same indications, uses, and side effects as described in NMOSD **(Table 1)**.

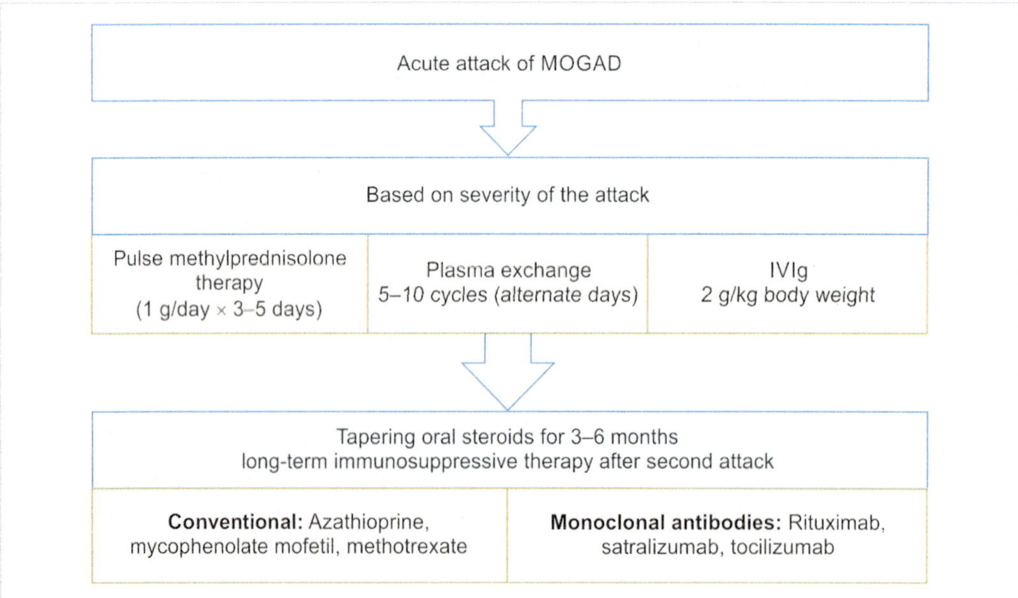

FLOWCHART 2: Management of MOGAD.

(IVIg: intravenous immunoglobulin; MOGAD: myelin oligodendrocyte glycoprotein antibody-associated disease)

Rituximab

Rituximab is a chimeric monoclonal antibody that targets CD20-positive B-cells and depletes them. It is US FDA approved for use in non-Hodgkin's lymphoma, chronic lymphocytic leukemia, rheumatoid arthritis, pemphigus vulgaris, and microscopic polyangiitis but is used off-label for many autoimmune and lymphoproliferative disorders including MOGAD. No RCTs on its use in MOGAD have been published, but data from retrospective review have shown long-term safety and efficacy in decreasing the annual relapse rate.[33,34] A systematic review and meta-analysis found that 55% of MOGAD patients remain relapse free with rituximab.[35] However, there has been an evolving concern about its efficacy in MOGAD, when compared to NMOSD in view of relapses while on treatment. Most patients who relapsed were found to have undetectable B-cell population which suggests that other mechanisms (in addition to B-cells) might also be responsible for the pathophysiology of its relapses.[36] Additionally, anti-MOG antibodies can also be continuously produced by long-lived plasma cells as they are CD20 negative and thereby resistant to rituximab. The choice between conventional immunosuppressants and monoclonal antibodies depends on the physician's discretion in the absence of RCTs, with the former being used for milder attacks and the latter for more severe attacks. The dosing schedule of the first induction dose and follow-up doses follow the same principle as in NMOSD.

Tocilizumab

Since a significant proportion (~50%) of MOGAD patients continue to relapse on rituximab, tocilizumab, and satralizumab (IL-6 inhibitors) are being increasingly used to treat MOGAD attacks. A recent study revealed no relapses in 10 MOGAD patients treated with tocilizumab.[37] RCTs are ongoing to test the safety and efficacy of rituximab and satralizumab in MOGAD.

Intravenous Immunoglobulin

Immunoglobulins play an important role in humoral immunity; so, IVIg treatment is expected to reflect exposure of the recipient to the collective donor antibodies against many antigens and infections. IVIg is used in the treatment of various autoimmune disorders and immunodeficiency states. The dose of IVIg is 2 g/kg body weight transfused as an intravenous infusion over 5 days in divided doses. A recent study of 39 MOGAD patients showed the utility of IVIg in treating different MOGAD phenotypes, leading to improvement in visual acuity and expanded disability status scale (EDSS) scores.[32] The authors concluded that IVIg might be an effective treatment for acute MOGAD attacks and relapses.[32] In another large retrospective review of 876 adult patients identified as MOGAD, 59 patients were treated with maintenance periodic IVIg.[38] There was a significant reduction in relapses. Although there is no defined dosing algorithm, initially 2 g/kg is given monthly for two to three doses and then reduced to 1 g/kg monthly, although lower doses like 0.4 g/kg monthly and intervals higher than 4 weeks have also been used after initial disease stability, albeit with a higher relapse risk.[38] This is potentially an effective treatment among patients failing conventional immunosuppressants. However, cost and availability limit its use.

CONCLUSION

The long-term immunomodulatory treatment of NMOSD and MOGAD rests on prevention of acute exacerbations and thereby reduce cumulative disability. Choice of therapy has widened for NMOSD in view of recently approved newer therapies. Although no definitive class I evidence is available, MOGAD treatment entails use of conventional immunosuppressive agents, IVIG or tocilizumab in selective patients. It is imperative to monitor patients while on immunosuppressive therapy and periodic follow-up is necessary to ensure compliance, safety and disease stability.

REFERENCES

1. Wingerchuk DM, Banwell B, Bennett JL, Cabre P, Carroll W, Chitnis T, et al. International consensus diagnostic criteria for neuromyelitis optica spectrum disorders. Neurology. 2015;85(2):177-89.
2. Banwell B, Bennett JL, Marignier R, Kim HJ, Brilot F, Flanagan EP, et al. Diagnosis of myelin oligodendrocyte glycoprotein antibody-associated disease: International MOGAD Panel proposed criteria. Lancet Neurol. 2023;22(3):268-82.
3. Lennon VA, Wingerchuk DM, Kryzer TJ, Pittock SJ, Lucchinetti CF, Fujihara K, et al. A serum autoantibody marker of neuromyelitis optica: distinction from multiple sclerosis. Lancet Lond Engl. 2004;364(9451):2106-12.
4. O'Connor KC, McLaughlin KA, De Jager PL, Chitnis T, Bettelli E, Xu C, et al. Self-antigen tetramers discriminate between myelin autoantibodies to native or denatured protein. Nat Med. 2007;13(2):211-7.
5. Cacciaguerra L, Flanagan EP. Updates in NMOSD and MOGAD Diagnosis and Treatment: A tale of two central nervous system autoimmune inflammatory disorders. Neurol Clin. 2024;42(1): 77-114.
6. Kümpfel T, Giglhuber K, Aktas O, Ayzenberg I, Bellmann-Strobl J, Häußler V, et al. Update on the diagnosis and treatment of neuromyelitis optica spectrum disorders (NMOSD) – revised recommendations of the Neuromyelitis Optica Study Group (NEMOS). Part II: Attack therapy and long-term management. J Neurol. 2024;271(1):141-76.
7. Waters P, Fadda G, Woodhall M, O'Mahony J, Brown RA, Castro DA, et al. Serial Anti-Myelin Oligodendrocyte Glycoprotein Antibody Analyses and Outcomes in Children With Demyelinating Syndromes. JAMA Neurol. 2020;77(1):82-93.
8. Cobo-Calvo A, Ruiz A, Maillart E, Audoin B, Zephir H, Bourre B, et al. Clinical spectrum and prognostic value of CNS MOG autoimmunity in adults: The MOGADOR study. Neurology. 2018;90(21): e1858-69.
9. Jarius S, Wildemann B. Aquaporin-4 antibodies (NMO-IgG) as a serological marker of neuromyelitis optica: a critical review of the literature. Brain Pathol Zurich Switz. 2013;23(6):661-83.
10. Levy M, Mealy MA. Purified human C1-esterase inhibitor is safe in acute relapses of neuromyelitis optica. Neurol Neuroimmunol Neuroinflamm. 2014;1(1):e5.
11. Li J, Bazzi SA, Schmitz F, Tanno H, McDaniel JR, Lee CH, et al. Molecular Level Characterization of Circulating Aquaporin-4 Antibodies in Neuromyelitis Optica Spectrum Disorder. Neurol Neuroimmunol Neuroinflamm. 2021;8(5):e1034.
12. Tahara M, Oeda T, Okada K, Kiriyama T, Ochi K, Maruyama H, et al. Safety and efficacy of rituximab in neuromyelitis optica spectrum disorders (RIN-1 study): a multicentre, randomised, double-blind, placebo-controlled trial. Lancet Neurol. 2020;19(4):298-306.
13. Kleiter I, Gahlen A, Borisow N, Fischer K, Wernecke KD, Wegner B, et al. Neuromyelitis optica: Evaluation of 871 attacks and 1,153 treatment courses. Ann Neurol. 2016;79(2):206-16.
14. Mealy MA, Mossburg SE, Kim SH, Messina S, Borisow N, Lopez-Gonzalez R, et al. Long-term disability in neuromyelitis optica spectrum disorder with a history of myelitis is associated with age at onset, delay in diagnosis/preventive treatment, MRI lesion length and presence of symptomatic brain lesions. Mult Scler Relat Disord. 2019;28:64-8.
15. Stellmann JP, Krumbholz M, Friede T, Gahlen A, Borisow N, Fischer K, et al. Immunotherapies in neuromyelitis optica spectrum disorder: efficacy and predictors of response. J Neurol Neurosurg Psychiatry. 2017;88(8):639-47.
16. Costanzi C, Matiello M, Lucchinetti CF, Weinshenker BG, Pittock SJ, Mandrekar J, et al. Azathioprine: tolerability, efficacy, and predictors of benefit in neuromyelitis optica. Neurology. 2011;77(7):659-66.
17. Laplaud DA, Casey R, Barbin L, Debouverie M, De Sèze J, Brassat D, et al. Comparative effectiveness of teriflunomide vs dimethyl fumarate in multiple sclerosis. Neurology. 2019;93(7):e635-46.
18. Pittock SJ, Lennon VA, McKeon A, Mandrekar J, Weinshenker BG, Lucchinetti CF, et al. Eculizumab in AQP4-IgG-positive relapsing neuromyelitis optica spectrum disorders: an open-label pilot study. Lancet Neurol. 2013;12(6):554-62.

19. Pittock SJ, Berthele A, Fujihara K, Kim HJ, Levy M, Palace J, et al. Eculizumab in Aquaporin-4-Positive Neuromyelitis Optica Spectrum Disorder. N Engl J Med. 2019;381(7):614-25.
20. Kim HJ, Nakashima I, Viswanathan S, Wang KC, Shang S, Miller L, et al. Eculizumab in Asian patients with anti-aquaporin-IgG-positive neuromyelitis optica spectrum disorder: A subgroup analysis from the randomized phase 3 PREVENT trial and its open-label extension. Mult Scler Relat Disord. 2021;50:102849.
21. Pittock SJ, Barnett M, Bennett JL, Berthele A, de Sèze J, Levy M, et al. Ravulizumab in Aquaporin-4–Positive Neuromyelitis Optica Spectrum Disorder. Ann Neurol. 2023;93(6):1053-68.
22. Traboulsee A, Greenberg BM, Bennett JL, Szczechowski L, Fox E, Shkrobot S, et al. Safety and efficacy of satralizumab monotherapy in neuromyelitis optica spectrum disorder: a randomised, double-blind, multicentre, placebo-controlled phase 3 trial. Lancet Neurol. 2020;19(5): 402-12.
23. Yamamura T, Kleiter I, Fujihara K, Palace J, Greenberg B, Zakrzewska-Pniewska B, et al. Trial of Satralizumab in Neuromyelitis Optica Spectrum Disorder. N Engl J Med. 2019;381(22): 2114-24.
24. Zhang C, Zhang M, Qiu W, Ma H, Zhang X, Zhu Z, et al. Safety and efficacy of tocilizumab versus azathioprine in highly relapsing neuromyelitis optica spectrum disorder (TANGO): an open-label, multicentre, randomised, phase 2 trial. Lancet Neurol. 2020;19(5):391-401.
25. Cree BAC, Bennett JL, Kim HJ, Weinshenker BG, Pittock SJ, Wingerchuk DM, et al. Inebilizumab for the treatment of neuromyelitis optica spectrum disorder (N-MOmentum): a double-blind, randomised placebo-controlled phase 2/3 trial. Lancet. 2019;394(10206):1352-63.
26. J Tullman M, Zabeti A, Vuocolo S, Dinh Q. Inebilizumab for treatment of neuromyelitis optica spectrum disorder. Neurodegener Dis Manag. 2021;11(5):341-52.
27. Marignier R, Bennett JL, Kim HJ, Weinshenker BG, Pittock SJ, Wingerchuk D, et al. Disability Outcomes in the N-MOmentum Trial of Inebilizumab in Neuromyelitis Optica Spectrum Disorder. Neurol Neuroimmunol Neuroinflamm. 2021;8(3):e978.
28. Aktas O, Smith MA, Rees WA, Bennett JL, She D, Katz E, et al. Serum Glial Fibrillary Acidic Protein: A Neuromyelitis Optica Spectrum Disorder Biomarker. Ann Neurol. 2021;89(5):895-910.
29. Fujihara K, Bennett JL, de Seze J, Haramura M, Kleiter I, Weinshenker BG, et al. Interleukin-6 in neuromyelitis optica spectrum disorder pathophysiology. Neurol Neuroimmunol Neuroinflamm. 2020;7(5):e841.
30. Carta S, Cobo Calvo Á, Armangué T, Saiz A, Lechner C, Rostásy K, et al. Significance of Myelin Oligodendrocyte Glycoprotein Antibodies in CSF: A Retrospective Multicenter Study. Neurology. 2023;100(11):e1095-108.
31. Macrini C, Gerhards R, Winklmeier S, Bergmann L, Mader S, Spadaro M, et al. Features of MOG required for recognition by patients with MOG antibody-associated disorders. Brain. 2021;144(8): 2375-89.
32. Lotan I, Chen JJ, Hacohen Y, Abdel-Mannan O, Mariotto S, Huda S, et al. Intravenous immunoglobulin treatment for acute attacks in myelin oligodendrocyte glycoprotein antibody disease. Mult Scler. 2023;29(9):1080-9.
33. Barreras P, Vasileiou ES, Filippatou AG, Fitzgerald KC, Levy M, Pardo CA, et al. Long-term Effectiveness and Safety of Rituximab in Neuromyelitis Optica Spectrum Disorder and MOG Antibody Disease. Neurology. 2022;99(22):e2504-16.
34. Durozard P, Rico A, Boutiere C, Maarouf A, Lacroix R, Cointe S, et al. Comparison of the Response to Rituximab between Myelin Oligodendrocyte Glycoprotein and Aquaporin-4 Antibody Diseases. Ann Neurol. 2020;87(2):256-66.
35. Nepal G, Kharel S, Coghlan MA, Rayamajhi P, Ojha R. Safety and efficacy of rituximab for relapse prevention in myelin oligodendrocyte glycoprotein immunoglobulin G (MOG-IgG)-associated disorders (MOGAD): A systematic review and meta-analysis. J Neuroimmunol. 2022;364:577812.
36. Kinzel S, Lehmann-Horn K, Torke S, Häusler D, Winkler A, Stadelmann C, et al. Myelin-reactive antibodies initiate T cell-mediated CNS autoimmune disease by opsonization of endogenous antigen. Acta Neuropathol (Berl). 2016;132(1): 43-58.
37. Elsbernd PM, Hoffman WR, Carter JL, Wingerchuck DM. Interleukin-6 inhibition with Tocilizumab for relapsing MOG-IgG associated disorder (MOGAD): A case series and review. Mult Scler Relat Disord. 2021;48:102696.
38. Chen JJ, Huda S, Hacohen Y, Levy M, Lotan I, Wilf-Yarkoni A, et al. Association of Maintenance Intravenous Immunoglobulin With Prevention of Relapse in Adult Myelin Oligodendrocyte Glycoprotein Antibody-Associated Disease. JAMA Neurol. 2022;79(5):518-25.

CHAPTER 6

Pediatric Demyelinating Disorders: Management Update

Lokesh Saini, Kandha Kumar UK

ABSTRACT

Pediatric acquired demyelinating syndromes (ADS) encompass a diverse array of immune-mediated diseases, including acute disseminated encephalomyelitis (ADEM), neuromyelitis optica spectrum disorders (NMOSD), myelin oligodendrocyte glycoprotein antibody-associated diseases (MOGAD), and multiple sclerosis (MS). Due to the overlapping and evolving nature of their symptoms, accurately distinguishing between these conditions based on initial presentation is complex. This chapter addresses the management strategies for these disorders, integrating recent evidence to guide treatment.

Keywords: Pediatric demyelinating disorders, ADEM, NMSOD, MOGAD, Management.

INTRODUCTION

Pediatric acquired demyelinating syndromes (ADS) include a broad spectrum of immune-mediated demyelinating diseases such as acute disseminated encephalomyelitis (ADEM), neuromyelitis optica spectrum disorders (NMOSD), myelin oligodendrocyte-glycoprotein antibody-associated diseases (MOGAD) and multiple sclerosis (MS). As the symptoms overlap and evolve over time, it becomes challenging to delineate the specific etiology based on the initial presentation. This chapter focuses on the management aspect of individual disorders in the context of recent evidence. **Figures 1 to 3** and **Table 1** depict the usual sites of involvement in various demyelinating disorders.[1]

MYELIN OLIGODENDROCYTE GLYCOPROTEIN ANTIBODY-ASSOCIATED DISEASE

Introduction

The common presentation of MOGAD includes ADEM (45.6%), optic neuritis (ON) (29.5%), transverse myelitis (TM) (11.2%), ON + TM (4.3%), and others (9.5%). Other rare forms of presentation include encephalitis-like phenotype, leukodystrophy-like phenotype, combined central and peripheral demyelination, overlapping syndromes, and nonclassifiable phenotypes.[2,3] Anterior segment ON/papillitis, conus involvement, and H-shaped spinal cord demyelination are strong clinico-radiological handles for early suspicion of MOGAD.

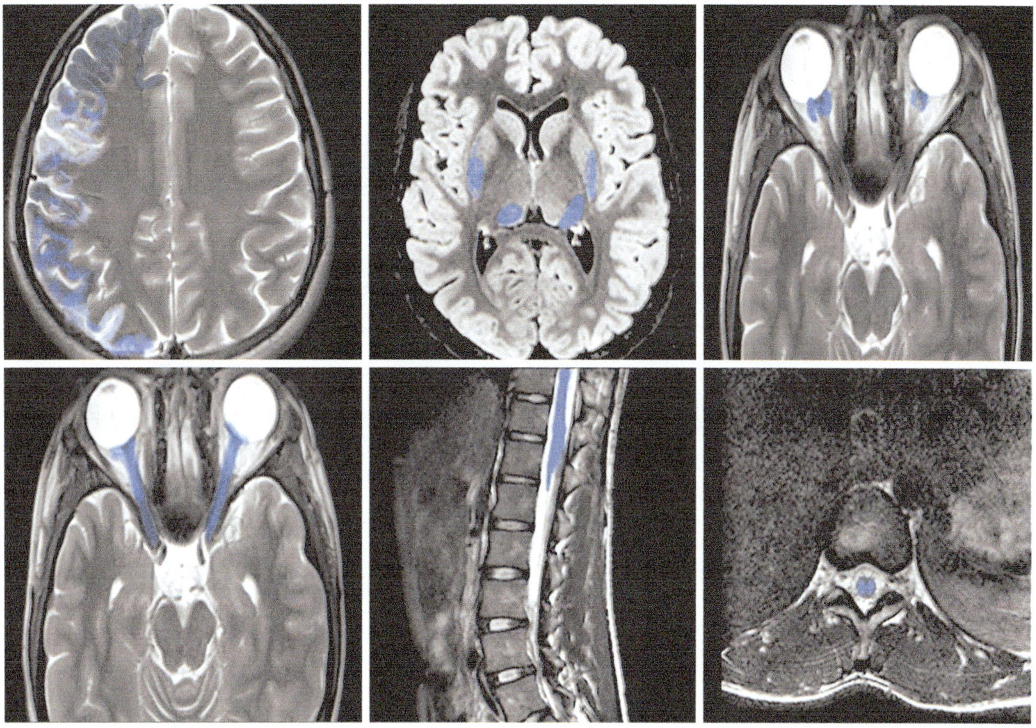

FIG. 1: Usual sites involved in myelin oligodendrocyte-glycoprotein antibody-associated diseases.

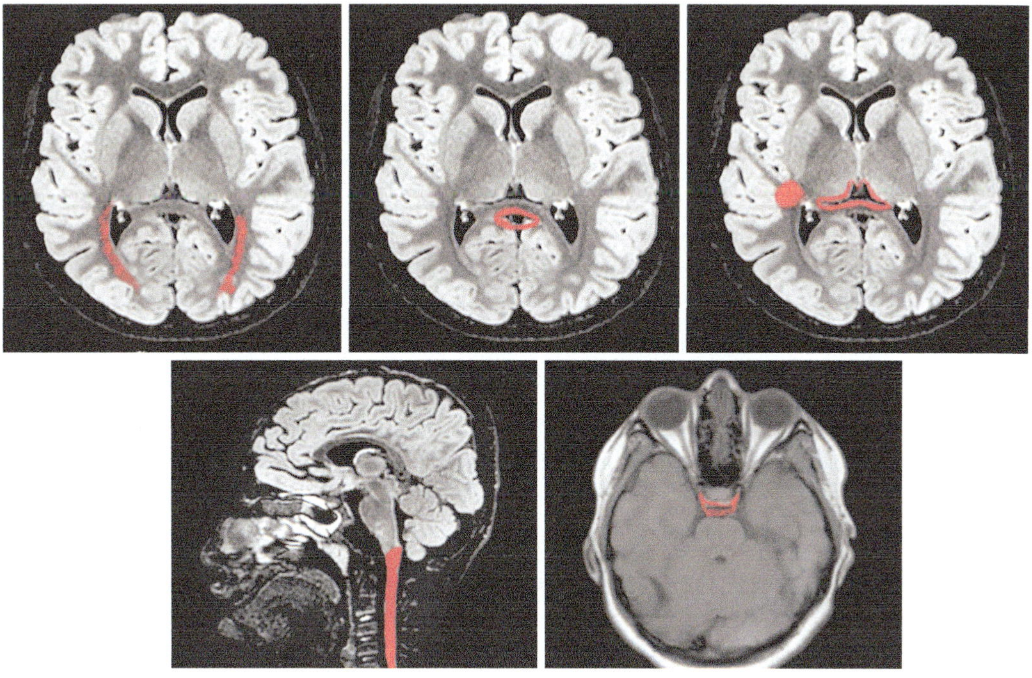

FIG. 2: Usual sites involved in neuromyelitis optica spectrum disorders.

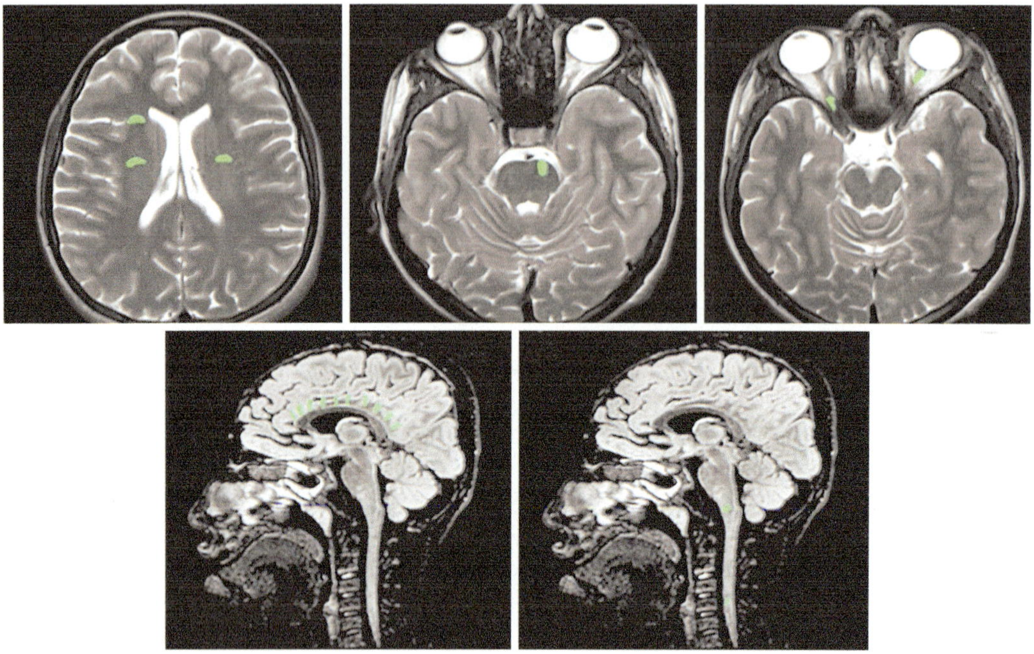

FIG. 3: Usual sites involved in multiple sclerosis.

TABLE 1: Usual sites involved in various demyelinating disorders.

Sites	MOGAD	NMOSD	MS
Brain	Small punctate to large tumefactive lesions in both white and deep gray matter;	Periaqueductal gray matter, area postrema, peri 4th ventricle, corticospinal tracts, rarely thalamus and brainstem	Ovoid lesion involving MS typical sites—juxtacortical, periventricular, and infratentorial. Ring-enhancing lesions are also commonly seen
Spine	Longitudinally extensive lesions involving >3 vertical segments, conus involvement, H-sign due to predominant gray matter involvement, and pencil-thin ependymal enhancement	Longitudinally extensive single lesion commonly involving the cervical cord. Holocord involvement in the axial images	Multiple short lesions; periphery of cord. Ring or nodular enhancement
Optic nerve	Long lesions in the anterior segments, papillitis, perineural sheath enhancement. Involvement can be unilateral or bilateral	Uni-/bilateral, mainly posterior segments, optic chiasma and optic tracts	Unilateral, short lesions, mainly involving the intraorbital portion

(MOGAD: myelin oligodendrocyte-glycoprotein antibody-associated diseases; NMOSD: neuromyelitis optica spectrum disorders; MS: multiple sclerosis)

Other variants of MOGAD include:

- Cortical—encephalitis-like phenotype;
- FLAMES (FLAIR-hyperintense lesions in anti-MOG-associated encephalitis with seizures);
- Leukodystrophy-like phenotype;
- Combined central and peripheral demyelination;
- Overlapping syndromes; and
- Pyrexia of unknown origin.

Pediatric versus Adult Myelin Oligodendrocyte Glycoprotein Antibody-associated Disease

Table 2 depicts the differences between pediatric and adult-onset MOGAD.[2-5]

Special Precautions in Pediatric Myelin Oligodendrocyte Glycoprotein Antibody-associated Disease

Children are more prone to infections following the immunotherapy. Screening for tuberculosis, retroviral infection, and viral hepatitis (hepatitis B and C) before initiating aggressive immunotherapy.

Prophylactic antibiotics including co-trimoxazole (5 mg/kg/day of trimethoprim component thrice a week) and fluconazole (3 mg/kg/day) should be started when children are treated with second-line immunotherapy like rituximab, tocilizumab, etc.

Table 3 depicts the vaccination schedule to be followed when children are on immunosuppressants.[6,7]

Treatment of Acute Attack

All acute attacks of MOGAD despite severity should be treated. Intravenous methylprednisolone (IVMP) at 20–30 mg/kg/day (maximum 1,000 mg) in a single dose for 5 consecutive days should be administered.[4,8-10] MOGAD generally has a very good response to steroids. However, the initial responsiveness to the glucocorticoids may neither necessarily prevent further relapses nor determine the severity and spectrum of clinical disease in further attacks.[4] In a large retrospective study, it was observed that IVMP caused complete resolution in 50% and partial response in 44% of the population.[11] IVMP should be followed

TABLE 2: Differences between pediatric and adult-onset MOGAD.

Characteristics	Pediatric MOGAD	Adult MOGAD
Incidence	0.31/100,000 children/year	0.13/100,000 adults/year
Prevalence among all ADS	35–40% of all pediatric ADS	5% of all ADS in adults
Most common presentation	ADEM like presentation	Optic neuritis and transverse myelitis
Incidence of relapses	Less common (Children <10 years old usually have a monophasic course. Incidence of relapse is 30–50% in children >10 years.)	More common (Incidence of relapse is 50–70% in adult patients)
Prognosis	Children <10 years old have more substantial recovery after the initial attack with a lower likelihood of relapse	Adolescents and adults especially those presenting with optic neuritis and transverse myelitis need long-term maintenance therapy

(ADS: acquired demyelinating syndromes; ADEM: acute disseminated encephalomyelitis; MOGAD: myelin oligodendrocyte-glycoprotein antibody-associated diseases)

TABLE 3: Recommendation for vaccination during immunosuppressant therapy.

Immunosuppressant therapy	Vaccination schedule
High dose prednisolone (2 mg/kg/day)	All vaccines can be administered 1 month after discontinuation of steroids
Moderated dose prednisolone (0.75–2 mg/kg/day)	No live vaccines until discontinuation of steroid therapy
Low dose alternate day steroids	Live vaccines can be administered concurrently
Treatment with rituximab	Avoid live vaccines until the CD-19 count recovers
Treatment with tocilizumab, cyclophosphamide	Avoid live vaccine until 3 months off therapy
Treatment with mycophenolate mofetil, azathioprine	Avoid live vaccine until 1 month off therapy

by oral prednisolone at 1-2 mg/kg/day for 4 weeks followed by tapering over 3 months. Slow tapering of oral steroids over 3-6 months may prevent relapses to a significant extent when compared to rapid tapering.[5,12]

If the Initial Intravenous Methylprednisolone Fails?

If the patient is refractory to the IVMP or shows inadequate response, therapeutic plasma exchange (TPE) should be initiated. A total of 5-7 sessions on every alternate day is recommended.[8] There are multiple studies demonstrating the benefits of TPE in patients who fail to respond to IVMP with complete recovery in 60-76% of the population.[5,11] Intravenous immunoglobulin (IVIg) at 2 g/kg over 2-5 days is an alternative in centers where TPE is not feasible.[8]

Maintenance Therapy

The usual course of MOGAD especially in the pediatric population tends to be monophasic with a very good response to initial treatment. The rationale for maintenance therapy is that, some degree of disability accumulates after each mild attack, increasing the likelihood of long-term morbidity.[13] There are no randomized controlled trials (RCTs) comparing the efficacy of individual immunosuppressants with one another. As per a recent systematic review, rituximab or IVIg can be used as the initial choice for maintenance therapy.[14,15]

Who are the Candidates for Maintenance Therapy?

- Patients with poor recovery after the initial attack defined by, Expanded Disability Status Scale (EDSS) ≥3, Modified Rankin Scale (MRS) ≥3, or visual acuity (VA) ≤0.3, even after 1-3 months of acute treatment.[8]
- Patients with clinical relapse.[8]

Parenteral Therapy

Intravenous Immunoglobulin

Monthly IVIg infusion as a maintenance therapy is also one of the efficacious methods to prevent relapse.[4,12] 1-2 g/kg over 1-5 days every month is recommended.[8] In a cohort study on pediatric MOGAD patients, annualized relapse rate (ARR) was lowest with IVIg when compared to all other maintenance immunosuppressants.[16] Adverse effects include headaches from aseptic meningitis and an increased risk of thromboembolic events. Subcutaneous immunoglobulin (SCIg) also has similar efficacy as that of IVIg and possesses cost-benefit.[17] However, studies are needed to validate its effect on MOGAD patients. Cost is an important limitation for its routine use.

Rituximab

Rituximab is a chimeric monoclonal antibody that targets CD20 on B cells and results in B-cell depletion. There are different protocols for dosing, frequency, and durations. The regimen usually followed in pediatric MOGAD is 375 mg/m^2/dose every week. Total of 2–4 doses is given by a standardized protocol. This cycle is repeated every 6 months. Monitoring of CD19 and 20 levels before the next dose is recommended. Common side effects are persistent hyperglobulinemia and leukopenia predisposing the patients for serious infections. Prophylactic antimicrobials such as co-trimoxazole and fluconazole may be considered. Despite adequate B-cell depletion, relapse occurs in about 25–86% of the population.[12,18-20]

Tocilizumab

Tocilizumab is an anti-interleukin-6 (IL-6) receptor monoclonal antibody, which is an important IL for B-cell maturation and antibody production. This is administered at a dose of 8 mg/kg through IV infusion every 4 weeks. It has been evaluated in retrospective observational studies for relapsing MOGAD. These studies, though limited in sample size, suggest that tocilizumab reduces ARR significantly.[21,22] However, potential adverse effects include increased infection risk, cytopenias, and elevated liver enzyme levels. Therefore, regular blood monitoring is essential, including a complete blood count and liver enzyme tests at baseline, monthly for the first 3 months, and every 2 months thereafter. Prophylactic antimicrobials such as co-trimaxazole and fluconazole may be considered.

The role of other immunosuppressants including cyclophosphamide, cyclosporin, mitoxantrone, or methotrexate in MOGAD is limited.

Oral Agents

Oral immunosuppressants including azathioprine and mycophenolate mofetil (MMF) are the preferred steroid sparing agents. Bridging therapy with low-dose prednisolone for 3–6 months is recommended, as these agents have an initial drug latency period to elicit immunosuppression.

Mycophenolate Mofetil

The MMF is the preferred oral immunosuppressant over azathioprine and its efficacy has been demonstrated in multiple cohort studies.[23-25] MMF elicits its immunosuppression by inhibiting inosine monophosphate dehydrogenase and thereby preventing T- and B-cell proliferation. The recommended dose is 600–1,200 mg/m^2/day (maximum 2 g/day) in two divided doses.[8] Adverse effects include gastrointestinal toxicity, risk of infections, and cytopenia. It should be used with caution in adolescent girls due to its potential risk for teratogenicity. Periodic monitoring of blood counts and liver function tests is mandatory.

Azathioprine

The recommended dose is 2–3 mg/kg/day in single or divided doses.[8] It is a purine synthesis inhibitor, thereby preventing B- and T- cell proliferation. Thiopurine-S-methyltransferase enzyme activity should be tested before initiating azathioprine as low enzyme activity cumulates the drug toxicity. Retrospective studies demonstrated the efficacy of azathioprine with a 50% reduction in relapse rates.[9,12,16] Adverse effects include infection, rash, transaminitis, bone marrow suppression, and risk of future malignancies. Periodic monitoring of blood counts and liver function tests is mandatory.

When to Withdraw the Maintenance Treatment?

Currently, there are no formal guidelines for the de-escalation and discontinuation of maintenance immunotherapy in MOGAD. Observations indicate that some patients experience long periods of stable disease without treatment and only relapse after several years, sometimes over a decade.

This suggests that continuous maintenance treatment over such extended periods may lead to overtreatment. Generally, it is advisable to consider de-escalating maintenance immunotherapy after 2 years of stable disease without relapses, along with stable visual, motor, autonomic, and cognitive assessments.[8]

Flowcharts 1 and 2 depict an overview on the management of MOGAD.

Special Considerations

Although there are no clear recommendations for the management of MOGAD variant, in children with ON or TM presentation long-term immunotherapy either with a low dose of prednisolone for 9–12 months or IV rituximab can be given. In children presenting with status epilepticus with uncontrolled raised intracranial pressure (ICP) and magnetic resonance imaging (MRI) showing cortical encephalitis, early initiation of second-line immunotherapy such as tocilizumab and TPE along with methylprednisolone can be considered.

NEUROMYELITIS OPTICA SPECTRUM DISORDERS

Introduction

Neuromyelitis optica spectrum disorder is an inflammatory disorder of the central nervous system, primarily affecting the spinal cord and optic nerves with involvement of other areas including the area postrema, periaqueductal gray matter, and hypothalamus. The disorder is known for its morbid attacks, chronicity, and a relapsing course. The clinical manifestations include ON, TM, area postrema syndrome, cerebral syndrome, acute brainstem syndrome, diencephalic clinical syndrome, and other overlapping autoimmune diseases.[26]

Management of Acute Attack

The treatment should be initiated immediately without any delay in NMOSD acute attacks. Acute therapy includes:

- IVMP, 30 mg/kg (maximum 1 g) for 3–5 days.

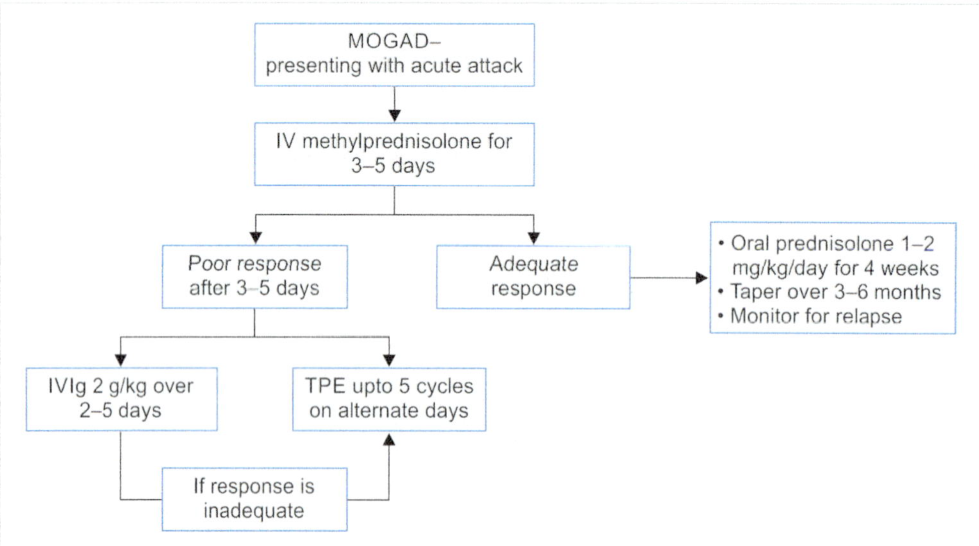

FLOWCHART 1: MOGAD—management of acute attack.

(IVIg: intravenous immunoglobulin; MOGAD: myelin oligodendrocyte-glycoprotein antibody-associated diseases; TPE: therapeutic plasma exchange)

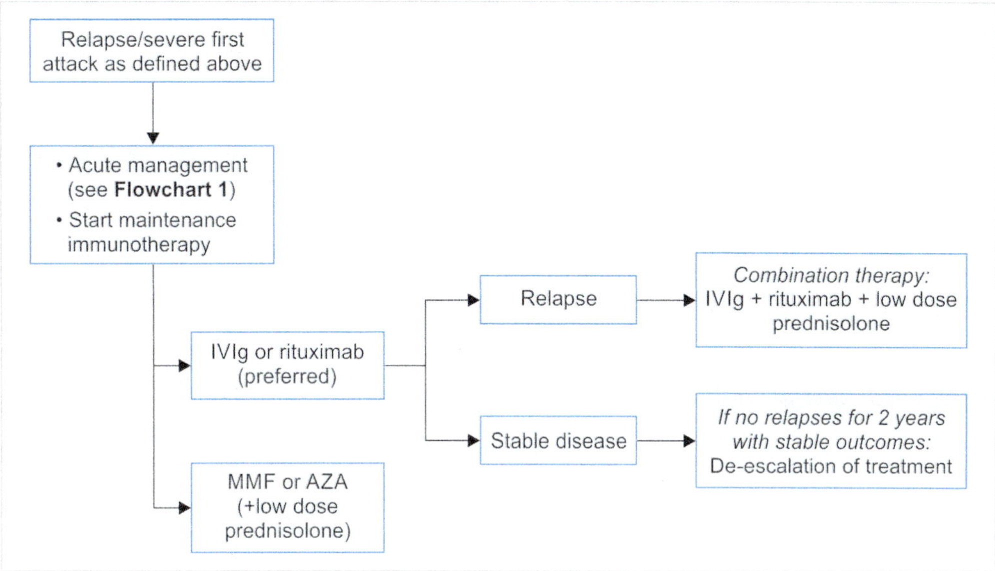

FLOWCHART 2: Maintenance therapy in MOGAD.
(IVIg: intravenous immunoglobulin, MMF: mycophenolate mofetil; AZA: azathioprine)

- If the patient shows insufficient response, then TPE 5–10 cycles on alternate days should be done.[27]
- In those patients, who showed insufficient response to steroids during previous attacks or sufficient response to apheresis therapy during previous attacks or those with severe myelitis, TPE is recommended as the first line treatment.[27]

Either plasma exchange or immunoadsorption may be used as apheresis therapy. For patients with severe attacks, concomitant treatment with IVMP and TPE may be used. This is followed by oral prednisolone at 1–2 mg/kg/day for 4 weeks and tapering over 3–6 months. However, the duration of oral steroids depends upon aquaporin 4 antibody-immunoglobulin G (AQP4-IgG) serostatus, disease activity, mode of action, and the expected time to the attack-preventive effect of the subsequent immunotherapy.

Flowchart 3 depicts the overview of the management of the initial attack of NMOSD.

Long-term Therapy

Indications: Long-term immunotherapy should be given to every patient with AQP4-IgG-positive NMOSD even after the first attack. The available treatment options include rituximab, IVIg, MMF, azathioprine, and upcoming future options include, tocilizumab, eculizumab, satralizumab, inebilizumab, and ofatumumab. The risk of recurrence of AQP4-IgG-positive NMOSD is 50% leading to disabling ON and TM.[28-30]

Rituximab

There are numerous studies demonstrating a significant reduction in annual relapse rates and even complete cessation of further relapses when rituximab is used as a maintenance therapy.[31,32] There are no standard protocols for dosing and frequency of rituximab administration. The commonly followed protocol is 375 mg/m^2/dose every week for 4 weeks. CD19 counts should be

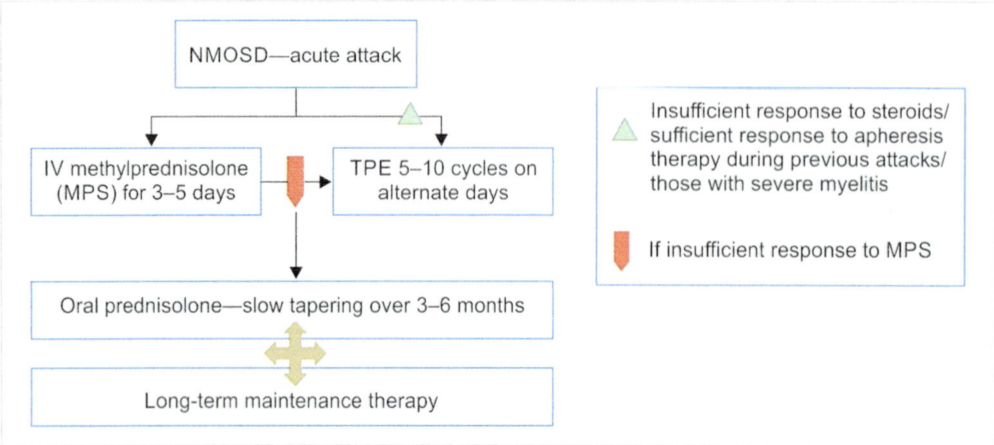

FLOWCHART 3: Overview of the management of the initial attack of NMOSD.

(IV: intravenous; IVMP: intravenous methylprednisolone; NMOSD: neuromyelitis optica spectrum disorders; TPE: therapeutic plasma exchange)

monitored 4 weeks after the last dose and then monthly. There is a higher chance of B-cell repopulation as early as 4 months following rituximab administration.[31] Further cycles are repeated every 6 months or when CD19 >1%.[33] Rituximab may be considered as a first-line maintenance therapy for relapse prevention in pediatric NMOSD patients.[34]

Intravenous Immunoglobulin

There are no studies to elucidate the role of IVIg in the pediatric NMOSD population as a long-term preventive therapy. A retrospective adult study showed a 66% reduction in relapse when IVIg is administered every 2 monthly.[35] Induction with 2 g/kg over 2–5 days during the acute attack followed by 1 g/kg/dose every month as maintenance therapy is recommended.

Mycophenolate Mofetil

The MMF is effective in pediatric NMOSD as a long-term preventive therapy. A large retrospective study showed that the median ARR and EDSS scores were significantly decreased, with 60% of patients being relapse-free.[24] The dose used is 600–1,200 mg/m^2/day in two divided doses. It should be overlapped with low-dose oral prednisolone for an initial 6 months. Periodic monitoring of blood counts and liver function tests is mandatory.

Azathioprine

Role of azathioprine was evaluated in a large cohort study containing both adult and pediatric population. It was found that reductions in relapse rate 89% and 61% remained relapse-free at 18 months after treatment initiation.[36] The recommended dose is 2–3 mg/kg/day in single or divided doses. Periodic monitoring of blood counts and liver function tests is mandatory.

New Treatment

Tocilizumab

There are two open-label studies in adult NMOSD patients showing the efficacy of tocilizumab as a preventive therapy.[37] There are few case reports in pediatric NMOSD, where tocilizumab provided a stable clinical course without relapse in rituximab failed patients.[38,39]

Future Treatments

Eculizumab

Eculizumab is a humanized monoclonal antibody designed to target the C5 complement protein, thereby inhibiting the alternate pathway of the complement cascade which attacks AQP4-expressing cells. Recently, the Food and Drug Administration (FDA) approved eculizumab for treating AQP4-IgG positive NMOSD in adult patients based on the phase 3 results of the PREVENT trial. It showed a relapse-free status in 98% of patients treated with eculizumab when compared to 63% of those receiving a placebo. However, its role in the pediatric population has not been validated.[34] One of the serious adverse effects of eculizumab is infection of capsulated organisms as membrane attack complex (MAC) is inhibited. Vaccination against pneumococcus, meningococcus, and *H. influenzae* should be done before the treatment.

Satralizumab

Satralizumab (SA237), similar to tocilizumab, is a humanized recombinant monoclonal antibody that targets the IL-6 receptor, offering immunomodulatory effects. In a phase 3 trial with 83 patients (composing 7 adolescent patients), satralizumab significantly lowered the risk of relapses, in the seropositive group.[40] Pediatric RCT is still in progress.

Inebilizumab

Inebilizumab is a humanized monoclonal antibody, targeted against CD19 B cells. It provides a broader depletion of B-cell lineage when compared to rituximab. In a phase 3 trial, with 230 adult patients with active NMOSD (93% seropositive), treatment with inebilizumab significantly reduced the risk of clinical relapses, disability progression, MRI lesion activity, and the need for hospitalizations compared to the placebo group. Experience in the pediatric population is not yet clear.

Duration of Long-term Therapy

There are no clear data, to recommend the duration and de-escalation of immunotherapy in NMOSD patients. Immunotherapy should be continued in stable AQP4-IgG-positive NMOSD patients, and must be closely monitored, if treatment is temporarily or permanently discontinued due to side effects or patient choice. In seronegative NMOSD patients who have been stable for over 5 years, reevaluation of immunotherapy may be considered.

ACUTE DISSEMINATED ENCEPHALOMYELITIS

The ADEM is a postinfectious demyelinating disorder of the central nervous system, triggered by an environmental stimulus (viral infection, vaccines) in genetically susceptible individuals.[41] The classic ADEM presents with acute febrile encephalopathy with multifocal neurological deficits, has a monophasic course, and responds well to immunotherapy.[42] Other variants include acute hemorrhagic leukoencephalitis, acute hemorrhagic encephalomyelitis, and acute necrotizing hemorrhagic leukoencephalitis of Weston Hurst.[43] As the most common presentation of MOGAD is an ADEM-like phenotype, serological testing for myelin oligodendrocyte glycoprotein (MOG) antibodies is recommended in all patients with suspicion of ADEM.[2]

Management

The initial management includes broad-spectrum antibiotics and acyclovir (until infective etiology is ruled out), antiraised ICP measures and seizure management. Once the possibility of ADEM is strongly considered, IVMP at 30 mg/kg/dose for 3–5 days is the initial treatment of choice.[44] This is followed by oral prednisolone at 1–2 mg/kg/day for 2 weeks followed by tapering over 4–6 weeks. If there is an inadequate clinical response to IVMP, TPE (in case of associated TM) or IVIg constitutes the second-line therapy.[44] Only patients with severe variants of ADEM will require second-line immunotherapy. For patients with a relapse of disease, we suggest intravenous (IV) glucocorticoids for acute management. There should be a careful review of the initial diagnosis for such patients to determine if their relapse represents multiphasic ADEM or another demyelinating syndrome such as MOG antibody-associated disease, MS, or NMOSD.

PEDIATRIC ONSET MULTIPLE SCLEROSIS

Multiple sclerosis characteristically being the disease of young adults, pediatric-onset MS (POMS) represents about 5% of total cases. The clinical course, management, and prognosis differ in the pediatric population. Relapsing-remitting multiple sclerosis (RRMS) is more common and constitutes about 97–99% of all POMS.[42,43]

Treatment of Acute Attack

Glucocorticoids remain the mainstay treatment for acute attacks. IVMP at 30 mg/kg/day for 3–5 days is the first-line treatment for an acute attack, followed by a short course of tapering oral steroids. If the patient relapses while tapering the steroid, either repeat IVMP or IVIg can be given. TPE is an alternative.

Disease-modifying Therapy for Pediatric-onset Multiple Sclerosis

The DMTs not only reduce the frequency of relapses but also decrease the T2 lesion load by targeting specific inflammatory elements that predominate during the relapsing-remitting course of MS. Nearly all DMT use in POMS, except fingolimod is off-label. Based on the results of the PARADIGMS trial comparing the efficacy of fingolimod versus interferon β-1a, FDA has approved oral fingolimod in children >10 years of age.[44] The dose is 0.25 mg once daily orally if weight is <40 kg and 0.5 mg once daily if weight is >40 kg. Adverse effects include bradycardia, cardiac arrhythmias, persistent lymphopenia, transaminitis, and basal cell carcinoma.[45]

There prevails a huge controversy between the use of escalation versus induction therapy. Considering the increased inflammatory load, young age at when the disability occurs, high relapse rates studies are favoring the initiation of high-efficacy early treatment (HEET) followed by maintaining on safer medications. In a recent observational study comparing the effectiveness of HEET (fingolimod, natalizumab, ocrelizumab, and alemtuzumab) versus medium efficacy treatment (MET) (interferon β-1a, glatiramer acetate, dimethyl fumarate, and teriflunomide) in POMS, it was found that patients starting with METs had much higher clinical disease activity than those initiated with HEET.[46]

Other DMTs approved in adult MS and which are under trial for pediatric use include

- *First-line DMTs*: Interferon β-1a, interferon β-1b, glatiramer acetate, and dimethyl fumarate.
- *Second-line DMTs*: Teriflunomide, natalizumab, alemtuzumab, cladribine, rituximab, and ocrelizumab.[47]

CONCLUSION

The clinical presentation, radiological hallmarks, treatment, and prognosis are distinct in pediatric-acquired demyelinating disorders. It is important to distinguish monophasic forms from relapsing phenotypes so that the use of chronic immunotherapy can be made more vigilant. MOG antibodies are detected in over 33% of all pediatric patients during the initial demyelination episode. AQP4 antibody positivity had high relapsing rates with significant long-term disability. Numerous clinical trials on novel therapeutic agents are in progress, and especially those on POMS are highly promising.

REFERENCES

1. Tillema JM. Imaging of central nervous system demyelinating disorders. Continuum (Minneap Minn). 2023;29(1):292-323.
2. Bruijstens AL, Lechner C, Flet-Berliac L, Deiva K, Neuteboom RF, Hemingway C, et al. E.U. paediatric MOG consortium consensus: Part 1 – Classification of clinical phenotypes of paediatric myelin oligodendrocyte glycoprotein antibody-associated disorders. Eur J Paediatr Neurol. 2020;29:2-13.
3. Waters P, Fadda G, Woodhall M, O'Mahony J, Brown RA, Castro DA, et al. Serial anti–myelin oligodendrocyte glycoprotein antibody analyses and outcomes in children with demyelinating syndromes. JAMA Neurol. 2020;77(1):82.
4. Hacohen Y, Wong YY, Lechner C, Jurynczyk M, Wright S, Konuskan B, et al. Disease course and treatment responses in children with relapsing myelin oligodendrocyte glycoprotein antibody–associated disease. JAMA Neurol. 2018;75(4):478.
5. Pandit L, Mustafa S, Nakashima I, Takahashi T, Kaneko K. MOG-IgG-associated disease has a stereotypical clinical course, asymptomatic visual impairment and good treatment response. Mult Scler J - Exp Transl Clin. 2018;4(3): 205521731878782.
6. Rao M IS, Kasi SG, Dhir SK, Wadhwa A, Rajsekhar B, Kumar CM, et al. Indian Academy of Pediatrics (IAP) Advisory Committee on Vaccines and Immunization Practices (ACVIP): Recommended Immunization Schedule (2023) and Update on Immunization for Children Aged 0 Through 18 Years. Indian Pediatr. 2024;61(2):113-25.
7. Papp KA, Haraoui B, Kumar D, Marshall JK, Bissonnette R, Bitton A, et al. Vaccination guidelines for patients with immune-mediated disorders on immunosuppressive therapies. J Cutan Med Surg. 2019;23(1):50-74.
8. Bruijstens AL, Wendel EM, Lechner C, Bartels F, Finke C, Breu M, et al. E.U. paediatric MOG consortium consensus: Part 5 – Treatment of paediatric myelin oligodendrocyte glycoprotein antibody-associated disorders. Eur J Paediatr Neurol. 2020;29:41-53.
9. Hacohen Y, Absoud M, Deiva K, Hemingway C, Nytrova P, Woodhall M, et al. Myelin oligodendrocyte glycoprotein antibodies are associated with a non-MS course in children. Neurol Neuroimmunol Neuroinflammation. 2015;2(2):e81.
10. Armangue T, Olivé-Cirera G, Martínez-Hernandez E, Sepulveda M, Ruiz-Garcia R, Muñoz-Batista M, et al. Associations of paediatric demyelinating and encephalitic syndromes with myelin oligodendrocyte glycoprotein antibodies: a multicentre observational study. Lancet Neurol. 2020;19(3):234-46.
11. Jarius S, Ruprecht K, Kleiter I, Borisow N, Asgari N, Pitarokoili K, et al.; in cooperation with the Neuromyelitis Optica Study Group (NEMOS) MOG-IgG in NMO and related disorders: a multicenter study of 50 patients. Part 2: Epidemiology, clinical presentation, radiological and laboratory features, treatment responses, and long-term outcome. J Neuroinflammation. 2016;13(1):280.
12. Ramanathan S, Mohammad S, Tantsis E, Nguyen TK, Merheb V, Fung VSC, et al. Clinical course, therapeutic responses and outcomes in relapsing MOG antibody-associated demyelination. J Neurol Neurosurg Psychiatry. 2018;89(2):127-37.
13. Lopez-Chiriboga AS, Sechi E, Buciuc M, Chen JJ, Pittock SJ, Lucchinetti CF, et al. Long-term Outcomes in Patients With Myelin Oligodendrocyte Glycoprotein Immunoglobulin G–Associated Disorder. JAMA Neurol. 2020;77(12): 1575.
14. Hennes EM, Baumann M, Lechner C, Rostásy K. MOG spectrum disorders and role of MOG-antibodies in clinical practice. Neuropediatrics. 2018;49(01):3-11.
15. Klein Da Costa B, Banwell BL, Sato DK. Treatment of MOG-IgG associated disease in paediatric patients: A systematic review. Mult Scler Relat Disord. 2021;56:103216.
16. Chen JJ, Flanagan EP, Bhatti MT, Jitprapaikulsan J, Dubey D, Lopez Chiriboga A (Sebastian) S, et al. Steroid-sparing maintenance immunotherapy for MOG-IgG associated disorder. Neurology. 2020;95(2): e111-20.
17. Perez EE, Orange JS, Bonilla F, Chinen J, Chinn IK, Dorsey M, et al. Update on the use of immunoglobulin in human disease: A review of evidence. J Allergy Clin Immunol. 2017;139(3):S1-46.
18. Albassam F, Longoni G, Yea C, Wilbur C, Grover SA, Yeh EA. Rituximab in children with myelin

oligodendrocyte glycoprotein antibody and relapsing neuroinflammatory disease. Dev Med Child Neurol. 2020;62(3):390-5.

19. Whittam DH, Cobo-Calvo A, Lopez-Chiriboga AS, Pardo S, Gornall M, Cicconi S, et al. Treatment of MOG-IgG-associated disorder with rituximab: An international study of 121 patients. Mult Scler Relat Disord. 2020;44:102251.
20. Durozard P, Rico A, Boutiere C, Maarouf A, Lacroix R, Cointe S, et al. Comparison of the response to rituximab between myelin oligodendrocyte glycoprotein and Aquaporin-4 antibody diseases. Ann Neurol. 2020;87(2):256-66.
21. Elsbernd PM, Hoffman WR, Carter JL, Wingerchuk DM. Interleukin-6 inhibition with tocilizumab for relapsing MOG-IgG associated disorder (MOGAD): A case-series and review. Mult Scler Relat Disord. 2021;48:102696.
22. Rigal J, Pugnet G, Ciron J, Lépine Z, Biotti D. Off-label use of tocilizumab in neuromyelitis optica spectrum disorders and MOG-antibody-associated diseases: A case-series. Mult Scler Relat Disord. 2020;46:102483.
23. Xu Y, Wang Q, Ren H tao, Qiao L, Zhang Y, Fei YY, et al. Comparison of efficacy and tolerability of azathioprine, mycophenolate mofetil, and cyclophosphamide among patients with neuromyelitis optica spectrum disorder: A prospective cohort study. J Neurol Sci. 2016;370: 224-8.
24. Huh SY, Kim SH, Hyun JW, Joung AR, Park MS, Kim BJ, et al. Mycophenolate Mofetil in the treatment of neuromyelitis optica spectrum disorder. JAMA Neurol. 2014;71(11):1372.
25. Montcuquet A, Collongues N, Papeix C, Zephir H, Audoin B, Laplaud D, et al. Effectiveness of mycophenolate mofetil as first-line therapy in AQP4-IgG, MOG-IgG, and seronegative neuromyelitis optica spectrum disorders. Mult Scler J. 2017;23(10):1377-84.
26. Tenembaum S, Yeh EA, The Guthy-Jackson Foundation International Clinical Consortium (GJCF-ICC). Pediatric NMOSD: A Review and position statement on approach to work-up and diagnosis. Front Pediatr. 2020;8:339.
27. Kümpfel T, Giglhuber K, Aktas O, Ayzenberg I, Bellmann-Strobl J, Häußler V, et al. Update on the diagnosis and treatment of neuromyelitis optica spectrum disorders (NMOSD) - revised recommendations of the Neuromyelitis Optica Study Group (NEMOS). Part II: Attack therapy and long-term management. J Neurol. 2024;271(1):141-76.
28. Flanagan EP, Cabre P, Weinshenker BG, Sauver JS, Jacobson DJ, Majed M, et al. Epidemiology of aquaporin-4 autoimmunity and neuromyelitis optica spectrum. Ann Neurol. 2016;79(5):775-83
29. Palace J, Lin DY, Zeng D, Majed M, Elsone L, Hamid S, et al. Outcome prediction models in AQP4-IgG positive neuromyelitis optica spectrum disorders. Brain. 2019;142(5):1310-23.
30. Kitley J, Waters P, Woodhall M, Leite MI, Murchison A, George J, et al. Neuromyelitis optica spectrum disorders with aquaporin-4 and myelin-oligodendrocyte glycoprotein antibodies: A comparative study. JAMA Neurol. 2014;71(3):276.
31. Nosadini M, Alper G, Riney CJ, Benson LA, Mohammad SS, Ramanathan S, et al. Rituximab monitoring and redosing in pediatric neuromyelitis optica spectrum disorder. Neurol Neuroimmunol Neuroinflammation. 2016;3(1):e188.
32. Longoni G, Banwell B, Filippi M, Yeh EA. Rituximab as a first-line preventive treatment in pediatric NMOSDs: Preliminary results in 5 children. Neurol Neuroimmunol Neuroinflammation. 2014;1(4):e46.
33. Cohen M, Romero G, Bas J, Ticchioni M, Rosenthal M, Lacroix R, et al. Monitoring CD27+ memory B-cells in neuromyelitis optica spectrum disorders patients treated with rituximab: Results from a bicentric study. J Neurol Sci. 2017;373:335-8.
34. Pittock SJ, Berthele A, Fujihara K, Kim HJ, Levy M, Palace J, et al. Eculizumab in aquaporin-4–positive neuromyelitis optica spectrum disorder. N Engl J Med. 2019;381(7):614-25.
35. Viswanathan S, Wong AHY, Quek AML, Yuki N. Intravenous immunoglobulin may reduce relapse frequency in neuromyelitis optica. J Neuroimmunol. 2015;282:92-6.
36. Elsone L, Kitley J, Luppe S, Lythgoe D, Mutch K, Jacob S, et al. Long-term efficacy, tolerability and retention rate of azathioprine in 103 aquaporin-4 antibody-positive neuromyelitis optica spectrum disorder patients: a multicentre retrospective observational study from the UK. Mult Scler J. 2014;20(11):1533-40.
37. Araki M, Matsuoka T, Miyamoto K, Kusunoki S, Okamoto T, Murata M, et al. Efficacy of the anti–IL-6 receptor antibody tocilizumab in neuromyelitis optica: A pilot study. Neurology. 2014;82(15):1302-6.
38. Breu M, Glatter S, Höftberger R, Freilinger M, Kircher K, Kasprian G, et al. Two Cases of pediatric aqp4-antibody positive neuromyelitis optica spectrum disorder successfully treated with tocilizumab. Neuropediatrics. 2019;50(03):193-6.
39. Marino A, Narula S, Lerman MA. First pediatric patient with neuromyelitis optica and sjögren syndrome successfully treated with tocilizumab. Pediatr Neurol. 2017;73:e5-6.

40. Yamamura T, Kleiter I, Fujihara K, Palace J, Greenberg B, Zakrzewska-Pniewska B, et al. Trial of satralizumab in neuromyelitis optica spectrum disorder. N Engl J Med. 2019;381(22):2114-24.
41. Stonehouse M. Acute disseminated encephalomyelitis: recognition in the hands of general paediatricians. Arch Dis Child. 2003;88(2):122-4.
42. Cole J, Evans E, Mwangi M, Mar S. Acute disseminated encephalomyelitis in children: an updated review based on current diagnostic criteria. Pediatr Neurol. 2019;100:26-34.
43. Waak M, Malone S, Sinclair K, Phillips G, Bandodkar S, Wienholt L, et al. Acute hemorrhagic leukoencephalopathy: pathological features and cerebrospinal fluid cytokine profiles. Pediatr Neurol. 2019;100:92-6.
44. Wang CX. Assessment and management of acute disseminated encephalomyelitis (ADEM) in the pediatric patient. Pediatr Drugs. 2021;23(3):213-21.
45. Boiko A, Vorobeychik G, Paty D, Devonshire V, Sadovnick D, the UBC MS Clinic Neurologists. Early onset multiple sclerosis: A longitudinal study. Neurology. 2002;59(7):1006-10.
46. Renoux C, Vukusic S, Mikaeloff Y, Edan G, Clanet M, Dubois B, et al. Natural history of multiple sclerosis with childhood onset. N Engl J Med. 2007;356(25):2603-13.
47. Chitnis T, Arnold DL, Banwell B, Brück W, Ghezzi A, Giovannoni G, et al. Trial of fingolimod versus interferon beta-1a in pediatric multiple sclerosis. N Engl J Med. 2018;379(11):1017-27.

CHAPTER 7

Newer Therapies in MS, NMOSD, and MOGAD

Bhawna Sharma, Madhuparna Paul

ABSTRACT

The spectrum of autoimmune inflammatory disorder of central nervous system (CNS) is expanding. There is a paradigm shift in the treatment of multiple sclerosis (MS), neuromyelitis optica spectrum disorder (NMOSD), and myelin oligodendrocyte glycoprotein antibody disease (MOGAD) over the last few decades that involves immune modulation, immune cell suppression or depletion, or enhanced immune cell sequestration. The present chapter provides an overview of therapeutic aspects of these autoimmune diseases.

Keywords: Multiple sclerosis, Relapsing remitting, AQP4, Myelin oligodendrocyte, Annualized relapse rate.

INTRODUCTION

Multiple sclerosis (MS), neuromyelitis optica spectrum disorder (NMOSD), and myelin oligodendrocyte glycoprotein antibody disease (MOGAD) are spectrum of autoimmune neurological disorder that involves brain and spinal cord. They cause demyelination and neurodegeneration characterized by inflammatory process that causes irreversible damage to central nervous system (CNS). Neuromyelitis optica (NMO) was initially described by Eugène Devic in the late 19th century as a variant of MS, presenting with optic neuritis and myelitis (Opticospinal MS). But the discovery of aquaporin-4 (AQP4) immunoglobulin G (IgG) antibody in 2004 proved that NMOSD is an astrocytopathy presenting with myelitis (short or long segment), optic neuritis, area postrema, diencephalic, brainstem, and symptomatic cerebral syndromes.[1,2] Some NMOSD patients, who are seronegative (around 20%),[3] have another antibody against myelin oligodendrocytes (MOG) in their serum and the clinical presentations include optic neuritis, myelitis, brainstem syndromes, acute disseminated encephalomyelitis (ADEM), or cortical encephalitis—an entity called MOGAD.

The prevention of attacks is recommended for all patients diagnosed with MS, NMOSD, and MOGAD, especially those with recurrent attacks. The aim is to avoid new attacks associated with the accumulation of neurological disabilities.

MULTIPLE SCLEROSIS

The disease-modifying treatments (DMTs) reduce inflammation, injury, neurodegeneration, and risk of relapses. Most drugs are

BOX 1: Types of multiple sclerosis (MS).

There are four categories of MS (Hauser and Goodin, 2005).

1. *Relapsing–remitting MS (RRMS)*: It is the most common type of MS (85%). There are relapses of symptoms and period of remission
2. *Secondary progressive MS (SPMS)*: The disease course continues to progress but may be associated with period of remission. It may be seen in some form of RRMS
3. *Primary progressive MS (PPMS)*: Here, the symptoms progressively worsen without any relapse or remission. Seen in around 10% patients, it is usually more resistant to treatment
4. *Progressive-relapsing MS (PRMS)*: Rarest form (<5%), progressive from beginning with outburst of worsening symptoms

Clinically Isolated syndrome: This is the first demyelinating episode which presents as optic neuritis or any cord or brainstem syndrome but does not fulfill the criteria for MS

BOX 2: Disease-modifying treatments (DMTs) in multiple sclerosis (MS).

Early "traditional" injectable DMT:

- *Interferon beta*:
- Glatiramer

FDA-approved oral agents:

- Sphingosine 1 phosphate modulator
- Teriflunomide
- Fumarates
- Cladribine

High-efficacy injectables and infusion:

- Natalizumab
- Rituximab
- Alemtuzumab
- Ocrelizumab
- Ofatumumab
- Mitoxantrone

Oral medicines under investigation:

- Bruton's tyrosin kinase inhibitor (BTKi)

Autologous hematopoietic stem cell transplantation

effective in relapsing remitting multiple sclerosis (RRMS) **(Box 1)**. There is a long list of DMTs evolved over the last three decades for the treatment of relapsing MS **(Box 2)**. It can be divided into low or moderate effective treatment agent (LETA), i.e., the first-line drugs (interferons, glatiramer, teriflunomide, and fumarates) and high-efficacy treatment agent (HETA) (S1P receptor modulators, natalizumab, anti-CD20 monoclonal antibodies, alemtuzumab, and cladribine), though the division is not equivocal. There are two strategies in MS treatment. One is escalation therapy where we start with conventional LETAs and monitor the response and shift to other LETA or HETA if the response is inadequate. Other is an evolving paradigm of induction therapy with early initiation of HETA. This reduces relapse rate and onset and progression of disability. The treatment of progressive MS is challenging with less response to immune-based therapy.[4]

Conventional Therapies

The conventional therapies for MS include interferon beta, glatiramer acetate, fingolimod, teriflunomide, fumarates , natalizumab, and mitoxantrone.

Cladribine

Approved by Food and Drug Administration (FDA) in 2019 for relapsing form of MS, it is a prodrug that is phosphorylated to the active metabolite cladribine 2-cholordeoxyadenosine triphosphate, causing intracellular accumulation of the metabolite hence disrupting cellular metabolism, DNA synthesis, and repair. CLARITY trial was a randomized, double-blind, and placebo-controlled trial that demonstrated a lower annualized relapse rate with cladribine compared to placebo. It is dosed by body weight (3.5 mg/kg), which is divided into two yearly treatment courses with two cycles per course that are spaced 1 month apart.

It carries an increased risk of malignancies, specifically benign uterine leiomyomas, melanoma, pancreatic, and ovarian carcinomas, so candidate needs to be selected with great caution.[5]

Injectables and Infusions

Alemtuzumab

Approved by FDA in 2014, it acts by binding to CD52, which is a cell surface antigen on T cells, B cells, monocytes, NK cells, and macrophages, causing antigen-dependent and complement-mediated cellular lysis. The recommended dose is two treatment cycles at 12 months interval, first cycle consisting of five infusions and the second cycle consists of three infusions. Alemtuzumab can cause secondary autoimmune disease (Graves' disease, immune thrombocytopenia, and antiglomerular basement membrane disease), malignancy (thyroid cancer, melanoma, and lymphoproliferative disorders), bone marrow suppression, and strokes. Higher serum IL-21 levels with higher T-cell apoptosis and cell cycling are responsible for secondary autoimmune diseases.[6]

Ocrelizumab

Approved by FDA in 2017 for RRMS, it is an intravenous humanized monoclonal antibody against anti-CD20 is also the only approved drug for primary progressive multiple sclerosis (PPMS). It acts by antigen-dependent and complement-mediated lysis of B cells. The OPERA I and OPERA II are two phase 3 multicentric double-blind studies comparing ocrelizumab with interferon beta 1a at 96 weeks showing reduction in annualized relapse rate and T1Gd-enhancing lesions. ORATORIO is the phase 3 trial showing significant reduction in disability progression at 24 weeks and T2 lesion volume in PPMS.[7]

Ofatumumab

Approved by FDA in 2020, ofatumumab is an injectable monoclonal antibody that binds to CD20+ B cells, causing B-cell depletion. It is used subcutaneously and has a shorter half-life and is immediately taken to the lymph nodes after the injection. Phase 2b MIRROR study showed 65% reduction in cumulative new Gd-enhancing magnetic resonance imaging (MRI) lesions compared to placebo at 12 weeks.[8] The ASCLEPIOS I and II were phase double-blind, double-dummy, randomized controlled trials showing lower relapse rates with ofatumumab compared to teriflunomide.[9]

Newly Emerging Oral Agents

Bruton's Tyrosine Kinase Inhibitors

They are emerging oral treatments for MS. Bruton's tyrosine kinases (BTKs) are Tec family tyrosine kinases that are expressed in B cells, monocytes, neutrophils, and mast cells and are important for B-cell maturation, proliferation, antigen presentation, and differentiation to plasma cells. In myeloid cells (monocytes and granulocytes), BTK is important for cytokine and inflammatory mediator production and phagocytosis. Evobrutinib, tolebrutinib, and orelabrutinib are CNS-penetrant Bruton's tyrosine kinase inhibitor (BTKi) and are shown to reduce T1 gadolinium-enhancing lesions in a dose-dependent manner in phase 2 trials. Several ongoing phase 3 clinical trials are underway and actively recruiting to investigate the efficacy of BTK inhibitors.[10]

Drugs in Pipeline for Multiple Sclerosis

Vidofludimus calcium (IMU-838) is a next-generation inhibitor of dihydroorotate dehydrogenase (DHODH), a mitochondrial enzyme that impairs DNA synthesis studied in a phase 2 trial in RMS and is in development in twinned, phase 3 studies in RRMS. Anakinra is recombinant interleukin receptor-1 antagonist, imatinib mesylate is an inhibitor of the Bcr-Abl tyrosine kinase, masitinib is a selective tyrosine kinase inhibitor targeting microglia and mast cells, foralumab (TZLS-401) is a human, anti-CD3 monoclonal antibody that modulates CD3 function, and SAR441344 is a monoclonal antibody that antagonizes the CD40 ligand, a costimulatory molecule of the immunologic synapse, are under study for RRMS. Belimumab, a B-cell-activating factor, is being developed as an add-on treatment to ocrelizumab in a phase 2 study of RMS. Ixazomib is a site-specific proteasome inhibitor that targets plasma cells that reduces CSF oligoclonal band (OCB) is under study.[11]

Remyelination and Neuroprotection in Multiple Sclerosis

It is a new strategy and an additional therapeutic approach in the field of MS. The effect of three neuroprotective medications (amiloride 5 mg, fluoxetine 20 mg, and riluzole 50 mg) is studied in UK in phase 2b, multiarm, double-blind, randomized, placebo-controlled trial on T2 lesion burden at 96 weeks, functional outcomes and time to first relapse in patients with SPMS, with no significant difference in the primary or secondary outcomes. A randomized, double-blind study using clemastine fumarate to target oligodendrocyte precursor differentiation demonstrated improvement in patients with RRMS and chronic demyelinating optic neuropathy.[12,13]

Metformin, a common medication used in diabetes mellitus, has been studied as a potential therapy to improve the regenerative potential of oligodendrocyte progenitor cells.[14]

Opicinumab, a monoclonal antibody targeting LINGO-1, a membrane protein that suppresses oligodendrocyte differentiation, was used in SYNERGY trial but was discontinued in a phase 2 trial due to not meeting primary and secondary endpoints.[14]

Progressive Multiple Sclerosis

The only current FDA-approved DMT for PPMS is ocrelizumab. Several other phase 3 clinical trials involving DMTs in the treatment of progressive (primary progressive and secondary progressive) MS have resulted in positive results. These include interferon beta (reduced disability progression), mitoxantrone, ocrelizumab, and siponimod. Several vitamins and cofactor such as biotin, lipoic acid, NAC, vitamin D supplementation have been studied for progressive MS. Cell-based therapy ATA188, an allogenic Epstein-Barr virus (EBV) T-cell therapy targeting EBV, which is well-recognized risk factor for MS, is underway.[1,12]

Microbiome

As different gut commensal can elicit pro-inflammatory and anti-inflammatory host responses, manipulating gut microbiota could be a therapeutic strategy for MS. Tauroursodeoxycholic acid (TUDCA) is a bile acid present in humans, a neuroprotective agent, an anti-inflammatory agent, and an apoptosis inhibitor. A phase 1/2 study in progressive MS is investigating the impact of TUDCA treatment on metabolomics, gut microbiota, and immunophenotyping. A single-arm, pilot study is investigating the safety and tolerability of oral fecal matter transplantation (FMT) in MS.[15]

NEUROMYELITIS OPTICA SPECTRUM DISORDER

The last decades witnessed the use of drugs, such as azathioprine (AZA), mycophenolate mofetil (MMF), tacrolimus, mitoxantrone, and cyclophosphamide, as off-label preventive treatments for NMOSD patients, with studies showing a reduction in annualized relapse rates.[16] The initial effect of AZA and MMF starts within 4-6 months; therefore, it is common to use oral corticosteroids as a bridging therapy for the initial treatment period. Another commonly used first-line therapy is rituximab (RTX), which requires intravenous infusions every 6 months, and the biological effect may be monitored by CD19+ cell count. RTX requires safety monitoring for immunoglobulin levels. RTX showed a greater association with relapse-free after long-term follow-up.

Tocilizumab (TCZ), a monoclonal antibody against the interleukin-6 (IL-6) receptor, has also been used as an off-label preventive treatment option for patients with NMOSD.[17] A comparative study with AZA [TCZ vs. azathioprine in NMOSDs (TANGO) study], TCZ was associated with a longer interval between attacks, as well as a reduction in the ARR.[18]

Eculizumab is a monoclonal antibody that blocks the complement protein C5 and prevents the activation of the complement cascade, in patients who were AQP4-IgG seropositive. The PREVENT trial (a randomized controlled trial of eculizumab in AQP4 antibody-positive participants with NMO) analyzed the efficacy of eculizumab and found it to be effective in reducing ARR in 94% of the patients when compared with placebo, and 98% of the patients were relapse free during a period of 12 months.[19]

Satralizumab is an IL-6 receptor blocker used in the treatment of NMOSD. SAkuraSky [Efficacy and Safety Study of Satralizumab (SA237) as add-on therapy to treat participants with NMO and NMO spectrum disorder] analyzed the effect of satralizumab, as an add-on therapy with AZA, MMF, and oral corticosteroids in patients with NMOSD.[20] In an RCT (SAkuraStar; Efficacy and Safety Study of Satralizumab), satralizumab was evaluated as a monotherapy for patients with NMOSD, both seropositive and seronegative, compared with placebo. Analysis suggests that satralizumab reduced the risk of relapse in seropositive AQP4-IgG.

Inebilizumab, a monoclonal antibody depleting CD19+ B cells, was compared with placebo in the N-MOmentum study (a clinical research study of inebilizumab in NMOSDs). Inebilizumab was associated with a reduced relapse risk in a period of 6 months.[21]

Ravulizumab is another humanized monoclonal antibody that binds to the same complement component C5 epitope as eculizumab. The CHAMPION-NMOSD study (an efficacy and safety study of ravulizumab in adult participants with NMOSD) selected only patients with seropositive AQP4-IgG NMOSD to receive treatment with ravulizumab and compared them with the placebo control group from the PREVENT study. All patients with AQP4-IgG-positive NMOSD treated with the ravulizumab group were relapse free.

Future perspectives:[22] An anti-CD20 monoclonal antibody, ublituximab, is being evaluated in combination with intravenous steroid for management of acute attacks in NMOSD patients. A preliminary phase 1 study showed a reduction in disability status over 90 days period.

Bortezomib, a 26S proteasome inhibitor approved for hematological neoplasms, was related to a relapse-free period of 12 months for four out of five patients with NMOSD and a decrease in AQP4-IgG levels.

Aquaporumab, a recombinant human monoclonal antibody against AQP4, was effective in reducing NMOSD lesions in in vitro models.

Bevacizumab, a humanized monoclonal antibody targets vascular endothelial growth factor A. It is currently being evaluated in a drug trial for the treatment in NMOSD.[23]

HBM9161 (HL161BKN), a human monoclonal antibody, acts by blocking neonatal Fc receptor (FcRn) and is currently under an open label dose exploration phase 1 trial.

Other therapies in pipeline are T4406F telitacicept (B-lymphocyte stimulator blocker and proliferation-inducing ligand), BTKi SHR1459 and DNA or T-cell vaccination, and the administration of AQP4 peptide loaded autologous tolerogenic dendritic cells. In a pilot trial, cetirizine, the antihistamine which blocks eosinophils, shows promising results as an add-on to other immunotherapies.[24]

Chimeric antigen receptor (CAR) T-cell therapy targeting B-cell antigens, such as CD19, is under investigation. A phase 1 trial in 12 AQP4-IgG-positive NMOSD patients showed no attacks in 11 patients during a follow-up of 5.5 months (median), but they have significant hematologic side effects. The generation of antigen-specific regulatory T cells (Treg) by transfection with T-cell receptors (TCRs) specific for particular autoantigens, aiming at antigen-specific tolerance induction. In Spain, in one phase 1b, open-label, multiple ascending doses, single-center clinical trial the safety and feasibility of tolerance-inducing dendritic cells (toldC)-based therapy has been investigated in NMOSD patients with good results.[25]

MYELIN OLIGODENDROCYTE GLYCOPROTEIN ANTIBODY DISEASE

About 50% of MOGAD has a monophasic course, so it is a matter of debate that whether all the patients will require maintenance treatment. Persistent MOG IgG seropositivity is associated with an increased risk of relapse. The adults are at a higher risk of relapse and may experience worse clinical outcomes than children.

The maintenance therapy for MOGAD has been extrapolated from NMOSD studies. Oral steroids, AZA, MMF, and B-cell-targeting biologics, such as RTX, and TCZ in addition to maintenance intravenous immunoglobulin (IVIg) can be used. Corticosteroids are associated with reduction in relapse rate, but the risk benefit ratio of prolonged corticosteroid use is to be kept in mind. When initiating AZA and MMF, it is recommended to bridge these patients with prednisolone for the first few months. RTX's efficacy in MOGAD patients remains ambiguous as there are no randomized clinical trials evaluating its effectiveness in this patient population. IVIg has emerged as a promising maintenance therapy for MOGAD patients. A multicentric retrospective cohort study conducted by Chen et al. reported that maintenance IVIg therapy was associated with a reduced relapse rate in adult MOGAD patients, especially when administered at a dose of 1–2 g/kg every 4 weeks. Other retrospective studies have suggested that maintenance IVIg therapy is effective in pediatric MOGAD patients also.[26,27]

Interleukin-6 inhibitors may play a role in MOGAD maintenance therapy with growing evidence suggesting that TCZ might be effective for highly relapsing MOGAD patients studied the effect of TCZ in annualized relapse rate decrease in patients with MOGAD and seropositive and seronegative AQP4-IgG NMOSD.[28]

B-cell-depleting monoclonal antibodies other than RTX, which have been studied in MOGAD, are ocrelizumab, ofatumumab, and anti-CD19 agent's inebilizumab.[29,30]

Eculizumab (anti-C5) that has been proven to be effective for relapse prevention in AQP4-IgG+NMOSD can be used in MOGAD, but very little data is available. Satralizumab is being investigated in a multicentric randomized clinical trials for MOGAD. Rozanolixizumab, an anti-neonatal Fc receptor inhibitor, is also a promising therapy that is currently in randomized clinical trials for the treatment of relapsing MOGAD patients.[31]

AUTOLOGOUS HEMATOPOIETIC STEM CELL TRANSPLANTATION

An emerging new therapy is autologous hematopoietic stem cell transplantation (AHSCT), which reset the immune. The aim is to destroy the aberrantly functioning immune system with high-dose chemotherapy and rebuild it with hematopoietic stem cell infusion, which induces long-term disease remission. There are four retrospective studies, five single-arm clinical trials, and two randomized control studies evaluating the efficacy of AHSCT in MS. The two randomized controlled trials were the ASTIMS and MIST trials proving the efficacy of AHSCT in MS. AHSCT seems to be a promising emerging therapy for MS, especially as a one-time treatment rather than long-term immunosuppression. The patients who seem to benefit most are those with lower disability at baseline, more active/relapsing disease, and younger ages, few or no comorbidities who have failed 1–2 high-efficacy DMTs.[32]

The evidence for AHSCT in NMOSD and MOGAD is limited and a proportion of patients will relapse within 5 years. Guidelines from the European Bone Marrow Transplantation (EBMT) Autoimmune Diseases Working Party (ADWP) recommend the use of AHSCT in NMOSD as an option, with grade II evidence, in therapy-refractory patients.[33] A recent meta-analysis includes three studies (published between 2000 and 2020) on 31 NMOSD patients who underwent AHSCT. Only one case report of a 25-year-old treatment-refractory male with MOGAD is found in the literature, who recovered very well after AHSCT.[34]

CONCLUSION

The last few decades have witnessed an expansion in the field of autoimmune diseases and so is the treatment. The advancements in the field of neuroimmunology have paved a new era for the treatment of these autoimmune neurological diseases with novel biologicals. However, the efficacy of the drugs is limited owing to their adverse effects. Further studies are required in this field to know the efficacy of these drugs and to identify the risk factors associated with these neuroinflammatory diseases, leading to neurodegeneration.

REFERENCES

1. Yang JH, Rempe T, Whitmire N, Dunn-Pirio A, Graves JS. Therapeutic Advances in Multiple Sclerosis. Front Neurol. 2022;13:824926.
2. Lennon VA, Wingerchuk DM, Kryzer TJ, Pittock SJ, Lucchinetti CF, Fujihara K, et al. A serum autoantibody marker of neuromyelitis optica: distinction from multiple sclerosis. Lancet. 2004;364(9451):2106-12.
3. Hamid SHM, Whittam D, Mutch K, Linaker S, Solomon T, Das K, et al. What proportion of AQP4-IgG-negative NMO spectrum disorder patients are MOG-IgG positive? A cross sectional study of 132 patients. J Neurol. 2017;264(10):2088-94.
4. Selmaj K, Cree BAC, Barnett M, Thompson A, Hartung HP. Multiple sclerosis: time for early treatment with high-efficacy drugs. J Neurol. 2024;271(1):105-15.
5. Giovannoni G, Comi G, Cook S, Rammohan K, Rieckmann P, Soelberg Sørensen P, et al.; CLARITY Study Group. A placebo-controlled trial of oral cladribine for relapsing multiple sclerosis. N Engl J Med. 2010;362(5):416-26.
6. Cohen JA, Coles AJ, Arnold DL, Confavreux C, Fox EJ, Hartung HP, et al.; CARE-MS I investigators. Alemtuzumab versus interferon beta 1a as first-line treatment for patients with relapsing-remitting multiple sclerosis: a randomised controlled phase 3 trial. Lancet. 2012;380(9856):1819-28.
7. Hauser SL, Bar-Or A, Comi G, Giovannoni G, Hartung HP, Hemmer B, et al.; OPERA I and OPERA II Clinical Investigators. Ocrelizumab versus Interferon Beta-1a in Relapsing Multiple Sclerosis. N Engl J Med. 2017;376(3):221-34.

8. Bar-Or A, Grove RA, Austin DJ, Tolson JM, VanMeter SA, Lewis EW, et al. Subcutaneous ofatumumab in patients with relapsing-remitting multiple sclerosis: The MIRROR study. Neurology. 2018;90(20):e1805-14. Erratum in: Neurology. 2018;91(11):538.
9. Hauser SL, Bar-Or A, Cohen JA, Comi G, Correale J, Coyle PK, et al; ASCLEPIOS I and ASCLEPIOS II Trial Groups. Ofatumumab versus Teriflunomide in Multiple Sclerosis. N Engl J Med. 2020;383(6): 546-57.
10. Haselmayer P, Camps M, Liu-Bujalski L, Nguyen N, Morandi F, Head J, et al. Efficacy and Pharmacodynamic Modeling of the BTK Inhibitor Evobrutinib in Autoimmune Disease Models. J Immunol. 2019;202(10):2888-906.
11. Cree BAC, Hartung HP, Barnett M. New drugs for multiple sclerosis: new treatment algorithms. Curr Opin Neurol. 2022;35(3):262-70.
12. Chataway J, De Angelis F, Connick P, Parker RA, Plantone D, Doshi A, et al. Efficacy of three neuroprotective drugs in secondary progressive multiple sclerosis (MS-SMART): a phase 2b, multiarm, double blind, randomised placebo-controlled trial. Lancet Neurol. 2020;19:214-25.
13. Green AJ, Gelfand JM, Cree BA, Bevan C, Boscardin WJ, Mei F, et al. Clemastine fumarate as a remyelinating therapy for multiple sclerosis (ReBUILD): a randomised, controlled, double-blind, crossover trial. Lancet. 2017;390:2481-9.
14. Neumann B, Baror R, Zhao C, Segel M, Dietmann S, Rawji KS, et al. Metformin restores CNS remyelination capacity by rejuvenating aged stem cells. Cell Stem Cell. 2019;25:473-85.e8.
15. Pröbstel AK, Baranzini SE. The Role of the Gut Microbiome in Multiple Sclerosis Risk and Progression: Towards Characterization of the "MS Microbiome". Neurotherapeutics. 2018;15(1): 126-34.
16. Shi M, Chu F, Jin T, Zhu J. Progress in treatment of neuromyelitis optica spectrum disorders (NMOSD): Novel insights into therapeutic possibilities in NMOSD. CNS Neurosci Ther. 2022;28:981-91.
17. Araki M, Matsuoka T, Miyamoto K, Kusunoki S, Okamoto T, Murata M, et al. Efficacy of the anti-IL-6 receptor antibody tocilizumab in neuromyelitis optica: a pilot study. Neurology. 2014;82(15):1302-6.
18. Digala L, Katyal N, Narula N, Govindarajan R. Eculizumab in the Treatment of Aquaporin-4 Seronegative Neuromyelitis Optica Spectrum Disorder: A Case Report. Front Neurol. 2021;12: 660741.
19. Kleiter I, Traboulsee A, Palace J, Yamamura T, Fujihara K, Saiz A, et al. Long-term Efficacy of Satralizumab in AQP4-IgG-Seropositive Neuromyelitis Optica Spectrum Disorder From SAkuraSky and SAkuraStar. Neurol Neuroimmunol Neuroinflamm. 2022;10(1):e200071.
20. Marignier R, Pittock SJ, Paul F, Kim HJ, Bennett JL, Weinshenker BG, et al.; N-MOmentum study investigators. AQP4-IgG-seronegative patient outcomes in the N-MOmentum trial of inebilizumab in neuromyelitis optica spectrum disorder. Mult Scler Relat Disord. 2022;57:103356.
21. Pittock SJ, Barnett M, Bennett JL, Berthele A, de Sèze J, Levy M, et al. Ravulizumab in Aquaporin-4-Positive Neuromyelitis Optica Spectrum Disorder. Ann Neurol. 2023;93(6):1053-68.
22. Sudhakar P, Abusamra K, Thandampallayam M, Kini A. New advancements in the management of Neuromyelitis Optica spectrum disease: literature review. Front. Ophthalmol. 2023;3:1130971.
23. Levy M. (2015). Efficacy of Bevacizumab (Avastin) in Treatment of Acute NMO Exacerbations. [online] Available from https://clinicaltrials.gov/ct2/show/NCT01777412?cond=NMO&draw=2&rank=9 [Last accessed September, 2024].
24. Zhu L-N, Hou H-M, Wang S, Zhang S, Wang GG, Guo ZY, et al. FcRn inhibitors: a novel option for the treatment of myasthenia gravis. Neural Regeneration Res. 2023;18(8):1637-44.
25. Derdelinckx J, Reynders T, Wens I, Cools N, Willekens B. Cells to the Rescue: Emerging Cell-Based Treatment Approaches for NMOSD and MOGAD. Int J Mol Sci. 2021;22:7925.
26. Chen JJ, Flanagan EP, Bhatti MT, Tisavipat N, Jamali S, Kunchok A, et al. Details and outcomes of a large cohort of MOG-IgG associated optic neuritis. Mult Scler Relat Disord. 2022;68:104237.
27. Lu Q, Luo J, Hao H, Liu R, Jin H, Jin Y, et al. Efficacy and safety of long-term immunotherapy in adult patients with MOG antibody disease: a systematic analysis. J Neurol. 2021;268(12):4537-48.
28. Elsbernd PM, Hoffman WR, Carter JL, Wingerchuk DM. Interleukin-6 inhibition with tocilizumab for relapsing MOG-IgG associated disorder (MOGAD): A case-series and review. Mult Scler Relat Disord. 2021;48:102696.
29. Graf J, Mares J, Barnett M, Aktas O, Albrecht P, Zamvil SS, et al. Targeting B Cells to Modify MS, NMOSD, and MOGAD: Part 1. Neurol Neuroimmunol Neuroinflamm. 2020;8(1):e918.
30. Graf J, Mares J, Barnett M, Aktas O, Albrecht P, Zamvil SS, et al. Targeting B cells to modify MS, NMOSD, and MOGAD: Part 2. Neurol Neuroimmunol Neuroinflamm. 2020;8(1):e919.

31. Sechi E, Cacciaguerra L, Chen JJ, Mariotto S, Fadda G, Dinoto A, et al. Myelin Oligodendrocyte Glycoprotein Antibody-Associated Disease (MOGAD): A Review of Clinical and MRI Features, Diagnosis, and Management. Front Neurol. 2022; 13:885218.
32. Burt RK, Balabanov R, Burman J, Sharrack B, Snowden JA, Oliveira MC, et al. Effect of Nonmyeloablative Hematopoietic Stem Cell Transplantation vs Continued Disease-Modifying Therapy on Disease Progression in Patients With Relapsing-Remitting Multiple Sclerosis: A Randomized Clinical Trial. JAMA. 2019;321(2): 165-74.
33. Sharrack B, Saccardi R, Alexander T, Badoglio M, Burman J, Farge D et al.; European Society for Blood and Marrow Transplantation (EBMT) Autoimmune Diseases Working Party (ADWP) and the Joint Accreditation Committee of the International Society for Cellular Therapy (ISCT) and EBMT (JACIE). Autologous Haematopoietic Stem Cell Transplantation and Other Cellular Therapy in Multiple Sclerosis and Immune-Mediated Neurological Diseases: Updated Guidelines and Recommendations from the EBMT Autoimmune Diseases Working Party (ADWP) and the Joint Accreditation Committee of EBMT and ISCT (JACIE). Bone Marrow Transplant. 2020;55:283-306.
34. Rush C, Atkins H. Aggressive and refractory MOG IgG Associated Encephalomyelitis Treated with Autologous Hematopoeitic Stem Cell Transplantation: First Case Worldwide. Mult Scler J. 2019;25:367-8.

CHAPTER

8

Switching Therapies in NMOSD and MOGAD

Suresh Kumar Radhakrishnan, Minu George

ABSTRACT

Neuromyelitis optica spectrum disorders (NMOSD) and myelin oligodendrocyte glycoprotein-associated disorders (MOGAD) are demyelinating diseases of the central nervous system, which have a relapsing course, and each attack can leave the patient with significant residual disabilities, especially if early therapy is not given.

Acute attacks must be treated early with high dose intravenous steroids. If the response is inadequate then quickly add on apheresis therapies or intravenous immunoglobulin (IVIg).

Long-term immune suppressive therapies to prevent subsequent attacks are the cornerstone of treatment. Drugs such as azathioprine, mycophenolate mofetil, and methotrexate are popular choices due to their easy availability and low cost. Long-term side effects are limiting factor in the use of these drugs. However, since the drugs have a long onset of action, bridging therapy with low-dose oral steroids is often given.

Rituximab, a B-cell depleter drug, is becoming increasingly popular in the treatment of especially NMOSD. This drug is again easily available, but one needs to be wary of the infusion related as well as long-term side effects due to immunosuppression of this drug.

Newer Food and Drug Administration (FDA)-approved drugs are the new kids in the block. They have a very specific and targeted mode of action and have shown good results in phase 3 trials. However, high cost may limit their use. Since most of these drugs have been very recently approved, their real-world data is lacking. However, these therapies show a lot of promise and may be the future armamentarium for physicians to get control of these disorders.

Keywords: Switch therapy, NMOSD, MOGAD.

INTRODUCTION

Switching of medications is common in the treatment of primary demyelinating diseases such as multiple sclerosis (MS), neuromyelitis optica spectrum disorders (NMOSD), and myelin oligodendrocyte glycoprotein antibody disease (MOGAD).

However, MS having a more frequent relapsing and remitting course, switching therapies is much more common than in NMOSD and myelin oligodendrocyte glycoprotein (MOG) disease. We know about 5–10% of NMOSD and 50% of MOG disorders are monophasic. In these disorders also, switching therapies may be done for a multitude of reasons. The most common being breakthrough disease in spite of compliance with treatment or intolerance of a particular drug due to adverse effects. However, high cost of therapy, family planning, pregnancy, preferences of patients, and aging are other situations wherein a switch might be required.

Switching can be a lateral switch between medications of similar efficacy due to intolerance or adverse effect of a drug. The other switch may be an escalation from a drug of lower to higher efficacy. Similarly, we may down escalate from a higher to a lower efficacy drug when infections or long-term side effects are a concern as in the case of risk of progressive multifocal leukoencephalopathy (PML) with natalizumab therapy in MS.

However, the decision when to switch from a particular therapy has never been easy. No uniform guidelines exist. There have been genuine attempts in this direction, but a well-accepted consensus across the various populations of the world is still elusive.

In this chapter, we attempt to look at various clinical scenarios where we may need a switch of therapy in NMOSD and MOG diseases. This includes both in the acute as well as long-term management of these diseases.

ACUTE RELAPSES IN NMOSD AND MOGAD: WHEN TO SWITCH EARLY

Acute attacks in both AQP4-IgG-positive and negative NMOSD are treated with high-dose glucocorticoids and plasma exchange (PE) therapy. Methylprednisolone (MP) should be administered intravenously (IV) at a dose of 1,000 mg/day for 3-5 days, followed by oral prednisolone. If the patient does not respond to MP within first few days, PE or immunoadsorption (IA) may be considered early **(Flowchart 1)**.[1-3] Six to ten cycles of apheresis may be considered based on improvement.[4] Several retrospective studies have shown that early apheresis therapy is associated with better outcomes in NMOSD patients. When apheresis therapy was started within 0–2 days of symptom onset without delay, up to 40% of patients showed complete remission; however, with a later

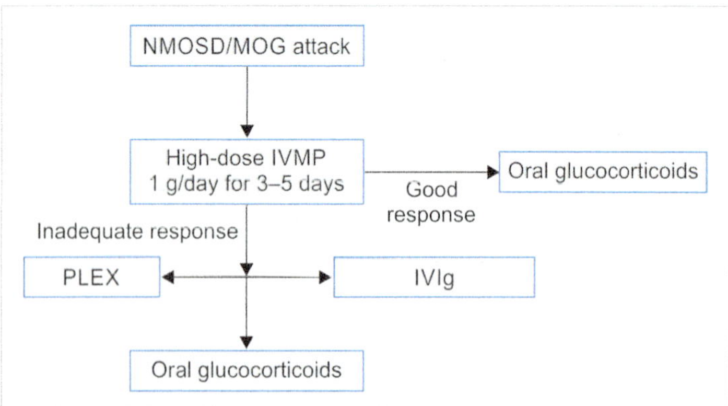

FLOWCHART 1: Switch therapy in acute NMOSD and MOGAD.

Note: Patient should initially be treated with high-dose IVMP for 3–5 days. In case of inadequate response to the same, option of PLEX/IVIg should be considered.

(IVIg: intravenous immunoglobulin; IVMP: intravenous methylprednisolone; MOG: myelin oligodendrocyte glycoprotein; MOGAD: myelin oligodendrocyte glycoprotein antibody disease; NMOSD: Neuromyelitis optica spectrum disorder; neuromyelitis optica spectrum disorder; PLEX: plasmapheresis)

treatment starting ≥7 days after symptom onset, only 3.7% of patients completely recovered.[5-7]

Usually, high-dose steroids are the first line of treatment, and in many centers, PE is considered a second-line or adjuvant therapy. However, the current opinion is to start PE as early as possible with steroids, especially when the patient does not show significant clinical improvement. PE and steroids are used concomitantly, especially in severe attacks involving the spinal cord and brain. Therapies used in acute treatment are shown in **Table 1**.[1-3]

The role of intravenous immunoglobulin (IVIg) in acute attacks needs more evidence. It is widely used in peripheral nerve disease such as Guillain-Barré syndrome and neuromuscular junction disorder such as myasthenia gravis, but its role in primary inflammatory disease of the central nervous system such as NMOSD is still lacking. However, there are small retrospective series where patients have benefitted from IVIg. Some experts in the field suggest the use of PE or IA as a first-line treatment option in the treatment for subsequent attacks, especially for longitudinally extensive transverse myelitis (LETM).[7,8]

Small case series also support the use of cyclophosphamide in acute steroid or PE-unresponsive NMOSD attacks, especially in the context of systemic lupus erythematosus (SLE) and other autoimmune diseases.[9,10]

In MOG-associated disorders, also known as MOGAD, treatment is very similar to NMOSD in its acute stage. Initially high-dose steroids (IVMP 1 g/day for 5 days) are given, and MOGAD with optic neuritis usually have a very good response. Both PE and immune-adsorption/apheresis therapy are used as rescue treatment.[11] IVIg is alternate second-line therapy in MOGAD, and it is particularly preferred in pediatric practice due to ease of use and tolerability. A dose of 1–2 g/kg/body weight over 5 days is preferred acute treatment regimen.[12]

SWITCH THERAPY WITH CONVENTIONAL DRUGS IN LONG-TERM MANAGEMENT OF NMOSD/MOGAD

The second main goal of NMOSD/MOGAD therapy is to prevent further attacks. Unlike MS, disability in NMOSD mainly results from poor and incomplete recovery from acute relapses.[3,7,13,14] AQP4-IgG-positive NMOSD typically takes a relapsing course, with high risk for attacks in the initial first year. Glucocorticoids, azathioprine, mycophenolate mofetil, or rituximab are commonly used as first-line agents for both AQP4-IgG-positive and -negative patients, with the reduction of attack rates irrespective of the serostatus in retrospective studies **(Table 2)**.

Rituximab is chimeric monoclonal antibody that binds to and deplete CD20-positive B cells. Its clinical efficacy has been demonstrated for both AQP4-IgG-positive

TABLE 1: Treatments used in acute relapses with their dose and side effect profile.

Treatment	Dose	Side effects
Methylprednisolone	1 g OD for 3–5 days	Hyperglycemia, hypertension, and insomnia
Plasmapheresis	6–10 cycles	Hypotension, hypocalcemia, bleeding diathesis, and GIT symptoms
IVIg	2 g/kg over 5 days	Infusion reaction, headaches, and liver and renal complications

(GIT: gastrointestinal tract; IVIg: intravenous immunoglobulin; OD: once daily)

TABLE 2: Major drugs used in chronic therapy of NMOSD/MOGAD.

Drug	Dose	Onset of action	Common side effects	Risk of infections	Blood monitoring
Azathioprine	1–3 mg/kg/day oral	6–12 months	Hematological abnormalities, elevation of liver enzymes, and increased risk of cancer (>10 years)	Respiratory and urinary infections and opportunistic infections	TC, DC, and liver enzymes
Mycophenolate mofetil	1,000–2,000 mg/day	8–12 weeks	Hematological abnormalities, elevation of liver enzymes, cancer, and teratogenic side effects	Respiratory and urinary infections and opportunistic infections	TC, DC, and liver enzymes
Glucocorticoids	Long term 7.5 mg/day	Immediate effects	Hematological, elevated liver enzymes, DM, hypertension, adrenal insufficiency, and Cushing's syndrome	Increased infections (PJP)	TC, DC, liver enzymes, and glucose levels
Rituximab	Premedicate with glucocorticoids and antihistamines. 1,000 mg 2 weeks apart followed by 500–1,000 mg every 6 months	B-cell depletion within 4 weeks and full onset of action after 8–12 weeks	Nausea, rashes, infusion-related pseudo allergic reactions (due to cell lysis), leukopenia, neutropenia, and hypogammaglobulinemia	Respiratory tract infections, allergic reactions, hepatitis B reactivation, and PML	TC, DC, and CD20 positive B cell count

(DC: differential count; DM: diabetes mellitus; MOGAD: myelin oligodendrocyte glycoprotein antibody disease; NMOSD: neuromyelitis optica spectrum disorder; PJP: *Pneumocystis jirovecii* pneumonia; PML: progressive multifocal leukoencephalopathy; TC: total count)

and -negative (adult and pediatric) patients in both prospective and retrospective studies with a reduction rate of over 80%.[15-17] A recent randomized double-blinded placebo trial from Japan also confirmed the efficacy of rituximab.[18] Most commonly followed schedule is 375 mg/m^2 body surface of IV every week for 4 weeks, followed by 6 months interval dosing. Most of the patients exhibit depletion of B cells in peripheral smear for at least 6 months after rituximab infusion; hence, redosing every 6 months should be ideal. Based on these trials, rituximab has been approved for treatment in Japan but widely used off-label in other countries.

The onset for B-cell depletion typically occurs in a few weeks; hence, CD19/20-positive B cells and CD27 memory cells can be used as surrogate markers for treatment monitoring and redosing.[19,20] Currently rituximab is considered the first-line drug for the management of this condition by many groups, while some others consider this a reserve drug when other common agents become ineffective.[21] The physician should take into account all patient-related factors and safety before starting treatment. Pre rituximab work-up includes hemogram, liver function tests, human immunodeficiency virus (HIV), hepatitis B surface antigen

(HBsAg), antihepatitis C antibody, antihepatitis B core antibody, and CD19/20 levels. The interleukin-6 (IL-6) receptor (IL-6R) antibody tocilizumab has also been increasingly used as a rescue therapy, showing benefits in several case series.[22]

The current guidelines[21,23] and expert opinion suggest azathioprine at a dose of 2.5–3 mg/kg as first-line therapy, accompanied by oral prednisolone 1 mg/kg/day or alternate day, slowly tapered after 2–3 months once azathioprine takes its clinical effect. Mycophenolate mofetil (MMF) is limited to persons where Azathioprine cannot be used.[21] However, there are experts who prefer MMF over azathioprine.

Switching among these groups of drugs is predominantly either due to side effect profiles or family planning/pregnancy or when escalation is a concern due to lack of efficacy. A switch due to intolerance of a drug, side effect profile, or pregnancy may be easier to decide. How ever it is difficult to decide when a switch is due to lack of efficacy. If a patient on conventional immunosuppressants, in spite being compliant and on adequate therapeutic doses, has a disabling relapse, switching to higher efficacious options as rituximab should be considered. MOGAD, being mostly a monophasic disease, the decision when to start long-term immunotherapy is debatable. Usually, clinicians prefer to start long-term immunomodulation after the second attack. Immunosuppression with corticosteroids, azathioprine, mycophenolate mofetil, methotrexate, etc., may be used.[24] In MOGAD, however it has been seen that rituximab may be less efficacious.

NEWER DRUGS IN THE TREATMENT OF NEUROMYELITIS OPTICA SPECTRUM DISORDER

Newer drugs, monoclonal antibodies that deplete CD19 B cells, inhibit complement protein C5 and IL-6 receptor blockade are currently being used in treatment of NMOSD **(Table 3)**.

TABLE 3: Newer drugs in treatment of NMOSD.

Drugs	Dose	Onset of action	Side effects	Risk of infections	Blood monitoring
Inebilizumab	IV with premeditations (glucocorticoids, antihistamines), initially 300 mg at day 1 and day 14, followed by 300 mg every 6 months	6–8 weeks	Arthralgia, back pain, infusion-related pseudoallergic reactions, lymphopenia, neutropenia, and hypogammaglobulinemia	Respiratory tract infection, urinary infection, and PML	TC, DC, and CD19/20 positive B-cell count
Eculizumab	IV 900 mg/ week 0–3 weeks, 1,200 mg in week 4, thereafter 1,200 mg every 2 weeks	Immediate within 1–2 weeks	Headache, anemia, leukopenia, fungal infections, and infusion-related reactions	Upper respiratory infections, and meningococcal infections	TC and DC

Continued

Continued

Drugs	Dose	Onset of action	Side effects	Risk of infections	Blood monitoring
Ravulizumab	IV, loading dose of 2,400–3,000 mg day 1, and 15 followed by 3,000–3,600 mg once every 8 weeks	Immediate in 1–2 weeks	Headache, anemia, leukopenia, and Infusion-related reactions	Upper respiratory infections, meningococcal infection, and fungal infection	TC and DC
Tocilizumab	IV 6–8 mg/kg/ body weight, every 4–6 weeks	After 12–24 weeks	Injection-related reactions, headache, neutropenia, thrombocytopenia, elevated liver enzymes, flare up of chronic diverticulitis with potential gastrointestinal perforations, elevation in cholesterol and triglycerides, and infusion-related allergic reactions	Respiratory infections and urinary infections	TC and DC
Satralizumab	120 mg at weeks 0, 2, and 4, followed by every 4 weeks	After 12–24 weeks	Injection-related reactions, headache, and arthralgia	Mild-to-moderate infections	TC, DC, liver enzymes, and lipid profile

(DC: differential count; IV: intravenous; MOGAD: myelin oligodendrocyte glycoprotein antibody disease; NMOSD: neuromyelitis optica spectrum disorder; TC: total count)

Inebilizumab

Inebilizumab is a humanized monoclonal antibody that binds and depletes CD19 positive B cells. The drug was approved for treatment in the United States in 2020 and in Europe in 2022. It is shown that B cells and plasma cells reduced to <10% of baseline, 4 weeks post-induction and to ≤4 cells/μL. Serum levels of glial fibrillary acidic protein (GFAP) and neurofilament light chain were significantly lower in patients treated with inebilizumab.[25]

Eculizumab

Eculizumab is a humanized monoclonal antibody that binds to complement protein C5 and disrupts the terminal complement cascade. The PREVENT trial showed that eculizumab as monotherapy or add-on therapy significantly reduced the risk of attacks.[26]

Ravulizumab

Ravulizumab is a long-lasting monoclonal antibody that targets the complement factor C5. Due to longer half-life, it needs to be administered only once in 8 weeks. The onset was rapid and near complete complement inhibition is observed after first infusion. To prevent opportunistic infections, patients should take meningococcal vaccine at least 2 weeks prior to starting drug.

Tocilizumab

Several studies have shown that IL-6R blockade with tocilizumab can prevent attacks in NMOSD.[27] Data on tocilizumab as first-line therapy for NMOSD is scare and hence not granted regulatory approval for NMOSD.[28]

Satralizumab

Satralizumab has been approved for treatment of AQP4-IgG-positive NMOSD in adults and adolescents aged 12 and older in Canada (2020), the United States (2020), Japan (2020), South Korea (2021), and Europe (2021). There is a limited experience using satralizumab as first-line therapy for adolescents with NMOSD.

AQP4-IGG-POSITIVE NMOSD: NEW DRUGS AND SWITCHING THERAPY

The efficacy of therapeutic antibodies in treating AQP4-IgG positive NMOSD is superior to classical immunosuppressants and makes them drugs of choice. A network meta-analysis on randomized controlled trial (RCT) data of these drugs suggests that complement inhibition with eculizumab may be more effective in preventing NMOSD attacks than treatment with inebilizumab and satralizumab.[29] The choice of first-line treatment for NMOSD relies on several factors such as disease activity and severity, mode and onset of action, possibility to combine with other immunosuppressive drugs, effect on autoimmune and other comorbidities, gender, frequency and route of administration, side effect, safety profile as well as drug availability, and approval status. Switching therapy depends on clinical improvement and further attacks **(Flowchart 2)**.

(*Note*: Patients should be first treated with rituximab, and in case of relapse, option of alternate treatment with newer monoclonal antibodies should be given to patient.)

SWITCH IN SPECIAL SITUATION/ FAMILY PLANNING/ PREGNANCY/ELDERLY

Neuromyelitis optica spectrum disorder can affect women with male-to-female ratio among AQP-IgG-positive patients of 1:10.[30] In 2020, therapeutic considerations on pregnancy-related treatment issues of NMOSD were published,[31] and a more detailed review on consensus-based recommendations on pregnancy and NMOSD was proposed by French MS society.[32] Factors

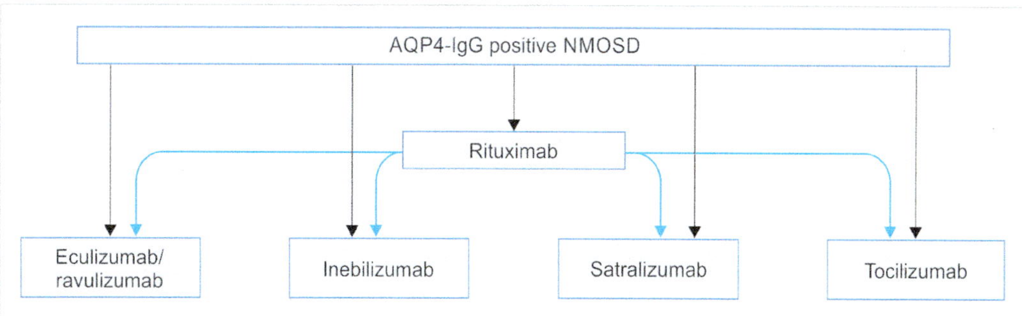

FLOWCHART 2: Switch therapy between rituximab and among newer drugs in adult NMOSD.
(IgG: immunoglobulin G; NMOSD: neuromyelitis optica spectrum disorder)

that increase the risk of disease activity during pregnancy include a positive AQP4-IgG serostatus, young age, disease activity before pregnancy, and withdrawal of immunotherapy.[33] Medications such as MMF and methotrexate are teratogenic and should be discontinued before pregnancy. It is found that monoclonal antibodies do not cross the fetoplacental barrier in first trimester but can transfer in second and third trimester. Azathioprine is relatively safe in NMOSD.[34] Female patients who are pregnant or planning to be pregnant while receiving eculizumab or ravalizumab may continue the therapy.[35] Tocilizumab has been used in pregnancy with rheumatoid arthritis and no increased risk of malformations has been reported.[36] Data on satralizumab and inebilizumab is very limited. Oral glucocorticoids may increase the risk of cleft palate if given in first trimester with increased risk of growth retardation and premature birth.[37] Though glucocorticoids can be administered with breast milk, breastfeeding should be delayed for 2–4 hours.[37] Methotrexate and mycophenolate should not be given during breastfeeding. Monoclonal antibodies are a viable option as the amount that transfers to mature breast milk is minimal.[38] In elderly, the risk of malignancy and infections are a matter of concern. Hence, drugs have to be selected very carefully keeping the high-risk profile in these populations under consideration.

PEDIATRIC NEUROMYELITIS OPTICA SPECTRUM DISORDER AND MYELIN OLIGODENDROCYTE GLYCOPROTEIN

Neuromyelitis optica spectrum disorder and MOGAD in adults and children can have similar symptoms, but there are some differences in the type of symptoms, their prevalence, and the treatments **(Table 4)**. AQP4-IgG seropositive patients have a greater than 50% risk of recurrence in the 12 months after diagnosis. Switching hence is more common in antibody-positive patients due to higher relapses. The clinical course of MOG-IgG-related disease is less clear, although initially reported to be typically monophasic, cumulative experience now suggests that, depending on published series, 25% to almost 75% will relapse, and some data suggests that this is particularly true if the serum MOG-IgG persists.[39] IVIg has more evidence in pediatric MOG than NMOSD.

TABLE 4: Pediatric NMOSD and MOGAD.

	NMOSD	MOGAD
Occurrence	3–5% of NMOSD cases	50% of MOGAD cases
Clinical features	Optic neuritis/transverse myelitis/ encephalopathy	ADEM/optic neuritis/transverse myelitis/ postpolar syndrome
Relapse rate	Lower in pediatric age	Lower in pediatric age
Functional recovery	Better in children	Better in children
Treatment	• *Acute*: IVMP/PLEX/IVIg • *Chronic*: Rituximab/mycophenolate/ azathioprine	• *Acute*: IVMP/PLEX/IVIg • *Chronic*: Azathioprine/mycophenolate/ rituximab/tocilizumab

(IVIg: intravenous immunoglobulin; IVMP: intravenous methylprednisolone; MOGAD: myelin oligodendrocyte glycoprotein antibody disease; NMOSD: neuromyelitis optica spectrum disorder; PLEX: plasmapheresis)

CONCLUSION

Switching therapies in NMOSD and MOGAD should be done based on age, efficacy, disease activity, side effects, availability, patients' choice, family planning, and cost. The earlier immunosuppressant therapies, though effective in many patients, were not backed by robust evidence-based clinical trials. Data on long-term management of these diseases is still lacking. There are no clear guidelines available as to when to switch therapies. However, if efficacy is not good and side effects are troublesome, then an early switch is indicated. Rituximab is currently a popular choice in NMOSD; however, its effect in MOGAD may be moderate at best. Newer Food and Drug Administration (FDA)-approved drugs are highly effective but costly. Their real-world data is also currently lacking. However, the clinicians now have a better armamentarium to tackle these diseases, which should augur well for the future.

REFERENCES

1. Bonnan M, Valentino R, Olindo S, Mehdaoui H, Smadja D, Cabre P. Plasma exchange in severe spinal attacks associated with neuromyelitis optica spectrum disorder. Mult Scler (Houndmills, Basingstoke, Engl). 2009;15:487-92.
2. Kleiter I, Gahlen A, Borisow N, Fischer K, Wernecke KD, Wegner B, et al. Neuromyelitis optica: evaluation of 871 attacks and 1153 treatment courses. Ann Neurol. 2016;79:206-16.
3. Siritho S, Nopsopon T, Pongpirul K. Therapeutic plasma exchange vs conventional treatment with intravenous high dose steroid for neuromyelitis optica spectrum disorders (NMOSD): a systematic review and meta-analysis. J Neurol. 2021;268:4549-62.
4. Padmanabhan A, Connelly-Smith L, Aqui N, Balogun RA, Klingel R, Meyer E, et al. Guidelines on the use of therapeutic apheresis in clinical practice—evidence-based approach from the writing committee of the American Society for Apheresis: the eighth special issue. J Clin Apher. 2019;34:171-354.
5. Bonnan M, Valentino R, Debeugny S, Merle H, Ferge JL, Mehdaoui H, et al. Short delay to initiate plasma exchange is the strongest predictor of outcome in severe attacks of NMO spectrum disorders. J Neurol Neurosurg Psychiatry. 2018;89:346-51.
6. Demuth S, Guillaume M, Bourre B, Ciron J, Zephir H, Sirejacob Y, et al. Treatment regimens for neuromyelitis optica spectrum disorder attacks: a retrospective cohort study. J Neuroinflamm. 2022;19:62.
7. Kleiter I, Gahlen A, Borisow N, Fischer K, Wernecke KD, Hellwig K, et al. Apheresis therapies for NMOSD attacks: a retrospective study of 207 therapeutic interventions. Neurol Neuroimmunol Neuroinflamm. 2018;5:e504.
8. Romeo AR. Segal BM. Treatment of neuromyelitis optica spectrum disorders. Curr Opin Rheumatol. 2019;31(3):250-5.
9. Saison J, Costedoat-Chalumeau N, Maucort-Boulch D, Iwaz J, Marignier R, Cacoub P, et al. Systemic lupus erythematosus-associated acute transverse myelitis: manifestations, treatments, outcomes, and prognostic factors in 20 patients. Lupus. 2015;24(1):74-81.
10. Yaguchi H, Sakushima K, Takahashi I, Nishimura H, Yashima-Yamada M, Nakamura M, et al. Efficacy of intravenous cyclophosphamide therapy for neuromyelitis optica spectrum disorder. Intern Med. 2013;52(9):969-72.
11. Sato DK, Callegaro D, Lana-peixoto MA, Waters PJ, Jorge FM, Takahashi T, et al. Distinction between MOG antibody positive and AQP4 antibody positive NMO spectrum disorders. Neurology. 2014;82:474-81
12. Bruijstens AL, Wendel EM, Lechner C, Bartels F, Finke C, Breu M, et al. EU paediatric MOG consortium consensus: Part 5—Treatment of paediatric myelin Oligodendrocyte Glyco-mprotein antibody associated disorders. Eur J Paediatric Neurol. 2020:29:41-53.
13. Jarius S, Ruprecht K, Wildemann B, Kuempfel T, Ringelstein M, Geis C, et al. Contrasting disease patterns in seropositive and seronegative neuromyelitis optica: a multicentre study of 175 patients. J Neuroinflamm. 2012;9:14
14. Molazadeh N, Filippatou AG, Vasileiou ES, Levy M, Sotirchos ES. Evidence for and against subclinical disease activity and progressive disease in MOG antibody disease and neuromyelitis

optica spectrum disorder. J Neuroimmunol. 2021;360:577702.

15. Dale RC, Brilot F, Duffy LV, Twilt M, Waldman AT, Narula S, et al. Utility and safety of rituximab in pediatric autoimmune and inflammatory CNS disease. Neurology. 2014;83:142-50.
16. Damato V, Evoli A, Iorio R. Efficacy and safety of rituximab therapy in neuromyelitis optica spectrum disorders: a systematic review and meta-analysis. JAMA Neurol. 2016;73:1342-48.
17. Dong GY, Meng YH, Xiao XJ. A meta-analysis on efficacy and safety of rituximab for neuromyelitis optica spectrum disorders. Medicine (Baltimore). 2022;101:e30347.
18. Tahara M, Oeda T, Okada K, Kiriyama T, Ochi K, Maruyama H, et al. Safety and efficacy of rituximab in neuromyelitis optica spectrum disorders (RIN-1 study): a multicentre, randomised, double-blind, placebo-controlled trial. Lancet Neurol. 2020;19:298-306.
19. Kim SH, Jeong IH, Hyun JW, Joung A, Jo HJ, Hwang SH, et al. Treatment outcomes with rituximab in 100 patients with neuromyelitis optica: influence of FCGR3A polymorphisms on the therapeutic response to rituximab. JAMA Neurol. 2015;72: 989-95.
20. Tahara M, Oeda T, Okada K, Ochi K, Maruyama H, Fukaura H, et al. Compassionate open-label use of rituximab following a randomised clinical trial against neuromyelitis optica (RIN-2 study): B cell monitoring-based administration. Mult Sclerosis Related Disorders. 2022;60:103730.
21. Sellner J, Boggild M, Clanet M, Hintzen RQ, Illes Z, Montalban X, et al. EFNS guidelines on diagnosis and management of neuromyelitis optica. Eur J Neurol. 2010;17:1019-32.
22. Ringelstein M, Ayzenberg I, Harmel J, Lauenstein AS, Lensch E, Stogbauer F, et al. Long-term therapy with interleukin 6 receptor blockade in highlyactive neuromyelitis optica spectrum disorder. JAMA Neurol. 2015;72:756-63.
23. Collongues N, de seze J. Current and future treatment approaches for neuromyelitis optica. Ther Adv Neurolo Disord. 2011;4:111-21.
24. Ramanathan S, Mohammad S, Tantsis E, Nguyen TK, Merheb V, Fung VS, et al. Clinical course, therapeutic response and outcomes in relapsing MOG antibody association demyelination. J Neurol Neurosurg Psychiatry. 2018;89:127-37.
25. Aktas O, Hartung HP, Smith MA, Rees WA, Fujihara K, Paul F, et al.; N-MOmentum study investigators. Serum neurofilament light chain levels at attack predict post-attack disability worsening and are mitigated by inebilizumab: analysis of four potential biomarkers in neuromyelitis optica spectrum disorder. J Neurol Neurosurg Psychiatry. 2023;94(9):757-68.
26. Pittock SJ, Berthele A, Fujihara K, Kim HJ, Levy M, Palace J, et al. Eculizumab in aquaporin-4-positive neuromyelitis optica spectrum disorder. N Engl J Med. 2019;381:614-25
27. Araki M, Matsuoka T, Miyamoto K, Kusunoki S, Okamoto T, Murata M, et al. Efficacy of the anti-IL-6 receptor antibody tocilizumab in neuromyelitis optica. Neurology. 2014;82:1302-6.
28. Zhang C, Zhang M, Qiu W, Ma H, Zhang X, Zhu Z, et al. Safety and efficacy of tocilizumab versus azathioprine in highly relapsing neuromyelitis optica spectrum disorder (TANGO): an open-label, multicentre, randomised, phase 2 trial. Lancet Neurol. 2020;19:391-401.
29. Wingerchuk DM, Zhang I, Kielhorn A, Royston M, Levy M, Fujihara K, et al. Network meta-analysis of food and drug administration-approved treatment options for adults with aquaporin-4 immunoglobulin G-positive neuromyelitis optica spectrum disorder. Neurol Ther. 2022;11:123-35.
30. Borisow N, Hellwig K, Paul F. Neuromyelitis optica spectrum disorders and pregnancy: relapse-preventive measures and personalized treatment strategies. EPMA J. 2018;9:249-56.
31. Mao-Draayer Y, Thiel S, Mills EA, Chitnis T, Fabian M, Katz Sand I, et al. Neuromyelitis optica spectrum disorders and pregnancy: therapeutic considerations. Nat Rev Neurol. 2020;16:154-70.
32. Vukusic S, Marignier R, Ciron J, Bourre B, Cohen M, Deschamps R, et al. Pregnancy and neuromyelitis optica spectrum disorders: 2022 recommendations from the French Multiple Sclerosis Society. Mult Scler (Houndmills, Basingstoke, Engl). 2023;29:37-51.
33. Kümpfel T, Thiel S, Meinl I, Ciplea AI, Bayas A, Hoffmann F, et al. Anti-CD20 therapies and pregnancy in neuroimmunologic disorders: a cohort study from Germany. Neurol Neuroimmunol Neuroinflamm. 2020;8:e913.
34. Meyer A, Drouin J, Weill A, Carbonnel F, Dray-Spira R. Comparative study of pregnancy outcomes in women with inflammatory bowel disease treated with thiopurines and/or anti-TNF: a French nationwide study 2010–2018. Aliment Pharmacol Ther. 2021;54:302-11.
35. Rondeau E, Ardissino G, Caby-Tosi MP, Al-Dakkak I, Fakhouri F, Miller B, et al. Pregnancy in women with atypical hemolytic uremic syndrome. Nephron. 2022;146:1-10.

36. Hoeltzenbein M, Beck E, Rajwanshi R, Gøtestam Skorpen C, Berber E, Schaefer C, et al. Tocilizumab use in pregnancy: analysis of a global safety database including data from clinical trials and post-marketing data. Semin Arthritis Rheum. 2016;46:238-45.
37. Boz C, Terzi M, Karahan SZ, Sen S, Sarac Y, Mavis ME. Safety of IV pulse methylprednisolone therapy during breastfeeding in patients with multiple sclerosis. Mult Scler J. 2018;24:1205-11.
38. LaHue SC, Anderson A, Krysko KM, Rutatangwa A, Dorsey MJ, Hale T, et al. Transfer of monoclonal antibodies into breastmilk in neurologic and non-neurologic diseases. Neurol Neuroimmunol Neuroinflamm. 2020;7:e769.
39. Tenembaum S, Yeh EA. Guthy-Jackson Foundation International Clinical Consortium (GJCF-ICC). Pediatric NMOSD: a review and position statement on approach to work-up and diagnosis. Front Pediatr. 2020;8:339.

CHAPTER

9

Management of Seronegative Central Nervous System Demyelinating Syndromes

Sruthi S Nair, Jemini George, Soumya Sundaram

ABSTRACT

The spectrum of central nervous system (CNS) demyelinating syndromes is widening. The most important non-multiple sclerosis (MS) demyelinating diseases are neuromyelitis optica spectrum disorders (NMOSD) and myelin oligodendrocyte glycoprotein-associated disease (MOGAD), both of which have pathognomonic autoantibodies. Despite using the best available assays, a significant proportion of non-MS demyelinating diseases do not yield any serological markers. This condition designated as "double seronegative" CNS demyelination may fulfil the consensus criteria for NMOSD or present as limited forms. The management of these patients is more challenging as they comprise a heterogeneous group and differ in many core characteristics from the seropositive population. There are few studies which have considered their clinicoradiological profile and fewer still assessing therapeutic response. Here, we review the available literature on the clinical presentation, diagnosis, and therapeutic approach toward double seronegative CNS demyelination.

Keywords: Double seronegative demyelination, NMOSD, Seronegative, Myelitis, Optic neuritis.

INTRODUCTION

Idiopathic inflammatory demyelinating disorders of central nervous system (CNS) comprise a heterogeneous group of disorders with diverse immunopathology. Multiple sclerosis (MS) is the most common and the best studied entity among them. Initially considered as a severe form of MS, neuromyelitis optica (NMO) emerged as a distinct entity with the discovery of antibodies to aquaporin-4 (AQP4) channels by Lennon et al. in 2004.[1] In the 2015 international consortium classification, the term NMO was extended to NMO spectrum disorder (NMOSD) acknowledging the brain lesions and site-restricted syndromes. This classification stratified the patients into seropositive and seronegative groups based on AQP4 immunoglobulin G (IgG) positivity.[2] In the next decade, several researchers demonstrated antibodies to myelin oligodendrocyte glycoprotein (MOG) in a subset of patients with seronegative NMOSD.[3] It soon became clear that these antibodies were also detectable among patients with other phenotypes such as acute disseminated encephalomyelitis (ADEM) and autoimmune meningoencephalitis earmarking MOG antibody-associated disease (MOGAD) as a separate disease.[4]

Patients presenting with a non-MS demyelinating syndrome and negative AQP4 and MOG antibodies in serum by a sensitive technique [cell-based assay (CBA)], are referred as having seronegative (or "double-seronegative") demyelinating disorders. A proportion of the double seronegative (DN) cases, ranging from 0 to 79% in various studies, fulfils the 2015 criteria for seronegative NMOSD.[5,6] Others may have site-restricted demyelination such as optic neuritis or myelitis, postinfectious demyelination, or less classical forms.[6] These seronegative demyelinating disorders represent a cluster of disparate diseases with unidentified antibodies and immune targets. They are, therefore, likely to have different recurrence risk and therapeutic responses compared to the classical seropositive group. In this review, we focus on the clinical and therapeutic aspects of the different seronegative demyelinating syndromes.

DOUBLE SERONEGATIVE DEMYELINATION FULFILLING CRITERIA FOR NEUROMYELITIS OPTICA SPECTRUM DISORDER

The pathophysiology of NMOSD is closely linked to antibodies against AQP4 water channels. The 2015 NMOSD diagnostic criteria defined a category of AQP4-seronegative or unknown status to facilitate treatment in resource-constrained settings and of the few true NMOSD patients where the antibody is persistently negative.[2] The criteria are more stringent than for AQP4-seropositve (AQP4-IgG+) patients. The diagnosis requires two of the six core diagnostic criteria of which at least one should be a classical presentation, namely, optic neuritis, myelitis, or area postrema syndrome. The less specific core criteria which include cerebral, brainstem, and diencephalic syndromes are not sufficient by themselves to fulfil the diagnosis. In addition, the additional magnetic resonance imaging (MRI) requirements typical for NMOSD should be met and alternative diagnosis for the symptoms should be excluded **(Box 1)**.[2]

It is now well accepted that MOGAD is a distinct disorder with different pathophysiology and treatment requirements and should not be considered as part of NMOSD.[5] Hence, only DN-NMOSD is truly considered among the seronegative category. Nearly 16% of appropriately phenotyped NMOSD patients were DN in a pivotal study.[7]

The clinical characteristics of DN-NMOSD patients are distinct from that of seropositive NMOSD and MOGAD. The DN cohort are generally younger and have an equal distribution of males and females compared to the female-dominant AQP4-IgG+ NMOSD.[6] Monophasic presentation and multifocal demyelination are more common. Several studies show higher frequency of simultaneous longitudinally extensive transverse myelitis (LETM) and optic neuritis. Myelitis and optic neuritis have been variably reported as the most common initial presentation.[6,8] Area postrema attacks are uncommon. In comparison to MOGAD, simultaneous bilateral optic neuritis or brain lesions are less common in DN-NMOSD.[6] Coexisting autoimmune diseases are less commonly observed in DN-NMOSD compared to AQP4-IgG+ NMOSD.[9]

In general, the severity of attacks and residual disability were similar in both seropositive and DN-NMOSD and both reached severe disability milestones nearly a decade earlier than patients with MOGAD.[10] Conversely, benign presentations may also be seen in the other end of the spectrum.[6] A large cohort from China showed milder attack severity and better prognosis for DN-NMOSD than AQP4-IgG+ NMOSD.[11] Relapsing disease occurs in 24–86% of patients in various studies.[6]

BOX 1: Categories of seronegative central nervous system demyelinating disorders.

1. Seronegative neuromyelitis spectrum disorder*

International consensus diagnostic criteria for seronegative NMOSD:

- At least two core clinical characteristics occurring from ≥1 clinical attacks and meeting all of the following requirements:
  - At least one core clinical characteristic must be optic neuritis, acute myelitis with LETM, or area postrema syndrome
  - Dissemination in space (two or more different core clinical characteristics)
  - Fulfillment of additional MRI requirements
- Negative tests for AQP4-IgG using best available detection method, or testing unavailable
- Exclusion of alternative diagnoses

Core clinical criteria:

- Optic neuritis
- Acute myelitis
- Area postrema syndrome
- Acute brainstem syndrome
- Acute diencephalic syndrome or narcolepsy
- Symptomatic cerebral syndrome with lesions typical of NMOSD

MRI criteria:

- *Acute optic neuritis:* MRI brain showing either normal or nonspecific findings *or* optic nerve MRI with T2-hyperintense lesion *or* T1-weighted contrast enhancing lesion extending over half the optic nerve length or involving optic chiasm
- *Acute myelitis:* Intramedullary MRI lesion extending over three or more contiguous segments *or* ≥3 contiguous segments of focal spinal cord atrophy in patients with remote history of myelitis
- *Area postrema syndrome:* Dorsal medulla/area postrema lesions
- *Acute brainstem syndrome:* Periependymal brainstem lesions

2. Limited forms of seronegative demyelination (monophasic or recurrent)

- Isolated atypical optic neuritis
- Isolated transverse myelitis (usually LETM)
- Hemispheric or brainstem syndromes with MS-atypical lesion(s)
- Acute disseminated encephalomyelitis (MOG negative)

(AQP4-IgG: aquaporin immunoglobulin G antibody; LETM: longitudinally extensive transverse myelitis; MOG: myelin oligodendrocyte glycoprotein; MRI: magnetic resonance imaging; MS: multiple sclerosis; NMOSD: neuromyelitis optica spectrum disorder)

*Criteria adapted from Wingerchuk DM, (2015).[2]

DOUBLE SERONEGATIVE DEMYELINATION WHICH DOES NOT SATISFY NEUROMYELITIS OPTICA SPECTRUM DISORDER CRITERIA

Seronegative demyelination with restricted presentation does not fulfil the consensus criteria for NMOSD and pose a more significant diagnostic challenge. Limited forms of DN demyelination commonly encountered include isolated atypical optic neuritis or isolated LETM. This rubric also includes brainstem syndromes and hemispheric tumefactive lesions with low lesion load. They may be monophasic or relapsing.[7] ADEM has MOG antibody positivity in 50% while the others are seronegative.[12]

Mimics of demyelinating disease such as sarcoidosis, connective tissue diseases, spinal cord ischemia, chronic infections such as tuberculosis and syphilis, metabolic disorders such as vitamin B12, folate, and vitamin E deficiency, copper deficiency, neoplasms, paraneoplastic myelopathy, and inherited disorders like Leber's hereditary optic neuropathy should always be considered in DN demyelination, particularly when poorly responsive to therapy or with other atypical features.[13,14]

TREATMENT

Data on therapy is less robust for DN demyelination than for AQP4 IgG+ NMOSD. The treatment includes management of acute attacks and preventive therapy. Most studies have shown comparable severity and residual weakness from an acute attack as for seropositive NMOSD and hence the therapeutic plan is generally similar. As there are no approved therapies in DN demyelination, maintenance therapy revolves around the use of broad-spectrum conventional immunosuppressants.[8] Some of the MS-specific disease modifying therapies, namely, interferon-β, glatiramer acetate, natalizumab, and fingolimod, can worsen NMOSD and should be ideally avoided in DN demyelination. Anti-CD20 agents are effective in both these situations.[6]

Acute Attacks

The standard of care for acute attacks is same in both seropositive and seronegative NMOSD.[15] The first line therapy is methylprednisolone which is administered intravenously at a dose of 1,000 mg/day for 3–5 days, followed by oral tapering dose (initiated at 1 mg/kg/day of prednisolone and tapered over 2–6 months). Inadequate recovery with methylprednisolone should prompt rapid escalation to rescue treatment with apheresis therapy such as plasma exchange (PLEX), usually five cycles every alternate day. Several studies have shown that early institution of PLEX within 1–2 days of symptom onset is associated with better outcomes compared to delayed treatment (≥7 days of onset) for seronegative NMOSD as well.[16,17] First-line treatment with PLEX may be considered in patients who had past history of poor response to glucocorticoids, previous good response to PLEX, and in severe myelitis.[15]

Prevention of Attacks

Disability in NMOSD mainly results from poor and incomplete recovery from clinical attacks.[18] Since monophasic episodes are more common in DN-NMOSD, the guidelines on initiation of maintenance immunotherapy are less lucid. Long-term immunotherapy in DN-NMOSD should be initiated after a second attack or after a severe first attack. A clear definition of "severe attack" is currently missing, and an attack is usually considered severe if a relevant functional deficit or impairment ensues.[15]

Currently there are no approved therapies for DN-NMOSD and treatment is guided by consensus. First-line treatments in DN-NMOSD include the conventional immunosuppressive therapies such as glucocorticoids, azathioprine, mycophenolate mofetil, and methotrexate. Rituximab can be optionally used as a first-line agent or when there is failure of first-line agents.[8] Cytotoxic agents such as parenteral cyclophosphamide, or mitoxantrone, are reserved for fulminant cases with poor response to the above agents **(Table 1)**.[19]

Four novel monoclonal antibodies, eculizumab, ravulizumab, inebilizumab, and satralizumab, have recently been approved for use in AQP4-IgG+ NMOSD.[20] Summary of evidence for newer agents in seronegative NMOSD is presented in **Table 2**. The N-MOmentum randomized controlled trial

TABLE 1: Maintenance immunotherapy in double seronegative demyelination.

Agent	Route	Dose	Side effects	Role
Prednisolone	Oral	1 mg/kg/day with tapering	Gastritis, hyperglycemia, hypertension, osteoporosis, hypokalemia, weight gain, sleep and mood disturbances, glaucoma, cataract	First-line, not preferred as monotherapy or long-term maintenance
Azathioprine	Oral	2–3 mg/kg/day (maximum 200 mg/day)	Bone marrow suppression, hepatic dysfunction, gastric adverse effects, rashes, infections, oncogenicity	First-line
Mycophenolate mofetil	Oral	2,000–3,000 mg/day	Gastrointestinal side effects, leukopenia, thrombocytopenia, hepatic dysfunction, infections, teratogenicity	First-line
Rituximab	IV	1,000 mg, two infusions over 2 weeks, repeated every 6 months	Infusion reactions, infections, hypogammaglobulinemia, progressive multifocal leukoencephalopathy (rare)	First or second line
Methotrexate	Oral	7.5–25 mg/weekly dose	Oral ulcers, gastroenteritis, alopecia, hepatic dysfunction, pneumonitis, interstitial lung disease	Alternate first-line
Cyclophosphamide	IV	750–1,000 mg every 1–2 months	Hemorrhagic cystitis, bone marrow suppression, infections, ovarian failure	Role in severe demyelination
Mitoxantrone	IV	12 mg/m^2 for 3–6 months	Gastrointestinal side effects, leukopenia, hair loss, ovarian failure, heart failure, leukemogenicity	Role in severe demyelination
Tocilizumab	IV	8 mg/kg every 4 weeks	Injection site reactions, infections, headache, cytopenia, hepatic dysfunction, dyslipidemia	Second or third line
Satralizumab	SC	120 mg on weeks 0, 2, and 4 and then every 4 weeks	Injection site reactions, thrombocytopenia, hepatic dysfunction dyslipidemia, infections	Second or third line
Inebilizumab	IV	300 mg 2 doses 2 weeks apart, then every 6 months	Infections, hypogammaglobulinemia, opportunistic infections	Second or third line

(IV: intravenous; SC: subcutaneous)

(RCT) of inebilizumab included both AQP4 IgG+ and seronegative NMOSD. Inebilizumab is an anti-CD19 agent with a broader range of immunosuppression than rituximab. The drug significantly reduced the risk of relapse in the combined group, however, the number of seronegative NMOSD was insufficient to deduce the utility in this group alone.[21]

Similarly, satralizumab, a monoclonal antibody targeting interleukin (IL)-6 receptor was studied in two placebo-controlled RCTs—SAkuraStar and SAkuraSky, both of which included AQP4 seropositive and negative patients. The number of seronegative patients were too small to derive an independent conclusion on efficacy in SAkuraStar,

TABLE 2: Clinical trials of novel immunotherapy in seronegative neuromyelitis optica spectrum disorder.

Therapeutic agent (trial)	Mechanism	Patient population (total, % SN)	Outcome in the whole group	Outcome in SN group
Tocilizumab (TANGO)	Anti IL-6 receptor	*TCZ*: 59, 15% SN *AZA*: 59, 10% SN	Relapse rate was 14% with TCZ vs. 47% in AZA	Relapse rate was 22% with TCZ vs. 50% in AZA
Satralizumab (SAkuraSky)	Anti IL-6 receptor	*SAT*: 41, 34% SN *PBO*: 42, 33% SN	Relapse rate was 20% with SAT vs. 43% with PBO	Relapse rate was 36% with SAT and 43% with placebo
Satralizumab (SAkuraStar)	Anti IL-6 receptor	*SAT*: 63, 35% SN *PBO*: 32, 28% SN	Relapse rate was 30% with SAT vs. 50% with PBO	Relapse rate was 46% with SAT vs. 33% with PBO
Inebilizumab (N-Momentum)	Anti CD19	*INB*: 174, 7.5% SN *PBO*: 56, 7% SN	Relapse rate was 12% with INB vs. 39% with PBO	Relapse rate was 17% with INB vs. 0 with PBO (very low sample size)

(AZA: azathioprine; IL-6: interleukin-6; INB: inebilizumab; PBO: placebo; SAT: satralizumab, SN: seronegative; TCZ: tocilizumab)

whereas, in SAkuraSky, the drug was deemed effective only in the seropositive group.[22,23] Satralizumab was continued alone or in combination with other immunosuppressive agents in the open label extension phase of the RCTs, where it was shown to be effective in both the groups in reducing the annualized relapse rate.[20]

The two complement inhibitor therapies, eculizumab and ravulizumab, were not studied in DN NMOSD in the pivotal RCTs, but isolated case reports have reported the benefit of the former in seronegative patients.[20]

Tocilizumab, another IL-6 receptor antagonist, has been reported to be efficacious in a phase 2 study and several case series and reports.[24,25] The phase 2 study of tocilizumab against azathioprine showed comparable efficacy in relapse reduction in seropositive and negative patients.[24] Though, a multitude of newer agents are under trials for NMOSD, few trials have allowed inclusion of seronegative NMOSD.

In case of recurrence of attack while on therapy, a combination of conventional agents or switching to tocilizumab or other novel monoclonal antibodies or experimental therapies may be considered. Experimental treatment includes intermittent PLEX or immunoadsorption or hematopoietic stem cell transplantation (HSCT).[15] **Flowchart 1** shows an algorithm for maintenance therapy in seronegative NMOSD.

As a single attack can result in significant disability, stopping immunotherapy is currently not recommended in AQP4-IgG+ patients. Data on treatment discontinuation in DN-NMOSD is scarce, however it may be considered in those who are stable for at least 5 years and have had only few and mild attacks.[15,26]

CONCLUSION AND FUTURE DIRECTIONS

Many gaps exist in the understanding and therapy of DN demyelination. Majority of the studies have focused on the antibody positive groups or evaluated NMOSD as a common cohort. Even more uncertainties remain in seronegative demyelination which fail to fulfil the consensus criteria for NMOSD. With the advances in fluid and radiological

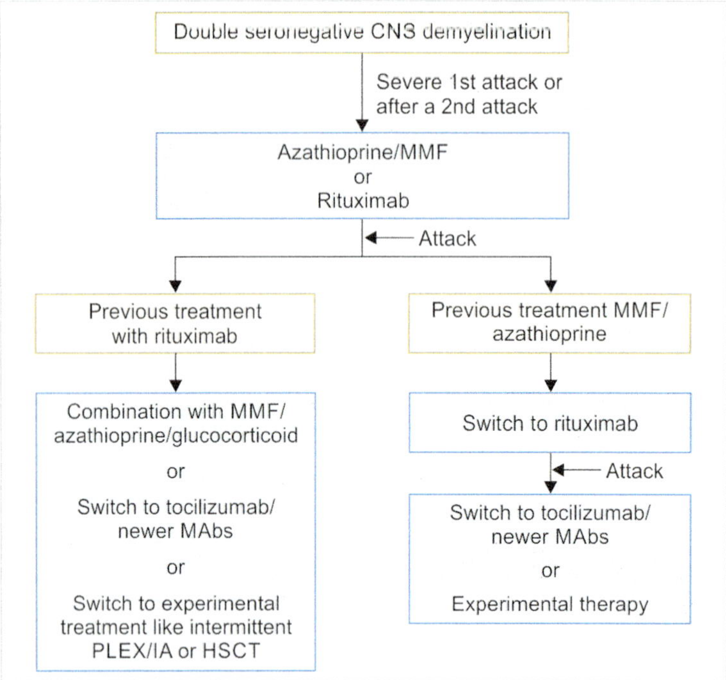

FLOWCHART 1: Algorithm for maintenance therapy in seronegative neuromyelitis optica spectrum disorders.

(CNS: central nervous system; HSCT: hematopoietic stem cell transplantation; IA: immunoadsorption: MAb: monoclonal antibody; MMF: mycophenolate mofetil; PLEX: plasma exchange)

biomarkers, it may be possible to evolve more uniform cohorts among DN demyelination and exclude the mimics. Trials on practical management of severe cases are also required to improve the strength of therapeutic guidelines.

REFERENCES

1. Lennon VA, Wingerchuk DM, Kryzer TJ, Pittock SJ, Lucchinetti CF, Fujihara K, et al. A serum autoantibody marker of neuromyelitis optica: distinction from multiple sclerosis. Lancet. 2004;364(9451):2106-12.
2. Wingerchuk DM, Banwell B, Bennett JL, Cabre P, Carroll W, Chitnis T, et al. International Panel for NMOD International consensus diagnostic criteria for neuromyelitis optica spectrum disorders. Neurology. 2015;85(2):177-89.
3. Ramanathan S, Reddel SW, Henderson A, Parratt JD, Barnett M, Gatt PN, et al. Antibodies to myelin oligodendrocyte glycoprotein in bilateral and recurrent optic neuritis. Neurol Neuroimmunol Neuroinflamm. 2014;1(4):e40.
4. O'Connell K, Hamilton-Shield A, Woodhall M, Messina S, Mariano R, Waters P, et al. Prevalence and incidence of neuromyelitis optica spectrum disorder, aquaporin-4 antibody-positive NMOSD and MOG antibody-positive disease in Oxfordshire, UK. J Neurol Neurosurg Psychiatry. 2020;91(10):1126-8.
5. Fujihara K. Neuromyelitis optica spectrum disorders: still evolving and broadening. Curr Opin Neurol. 2019;32(3):385-94.
6. Wu Y, Geraldes R, Juryńczyk M, Palace J. Double-negative neuromyelitis optica spectrum disorder. Mult Scler. 2023;29(11-12):1353-62.
7. Hamid SHM, Whittam D, Mutch K, Linaker S, Solomon T, Das K, et al. What proportion of AQP4-

IgG-negative NMO spectrum disorder patients are MOG-IgG positive? A cross sectional study of 132 patients. J. Neurol. 2017;264(10):2088-94.

8. Marin CE, Sato DK. Recent Advances on the Diagnosis and Management of Seronegative Neuromyelitis Optica Spectrum Disorder. touchREVIEWS in Neurology. 2024;20(1):10-5.
9. Schmetzer O, Lakin E, Roediger B, Duchow A, Asseyer S, Paul F, et al. Anti-aquaporin 4 IgG Is Not Associated With Any Clinical Disease Characteristics in Neuromyelitis Optica Spectrum Disorder. Front Neurol. 2021;12:635419.
10. Duchow A, Bellmann-Strobl J, Friede T, Aktas O, Angstwurm K, Ayzenberg I, et al. Time to Disability Milestones and Annualized Relapse Rates in NMOSD and MOGAD. Ann Neurol. 2024;95(4): 720-32.
11. Du Q, Shi Z, Chen H, Zhang Y, Wang J, Qiu Y, et al. Comparison of clinical characteristics and prognoses in patients with different AQP4-Ab and MOG-Ab serostatus with neuromyelitis optica spectrum disorders. J Neuroimmunol. 2021;353:577494.
12. Otallah S. Acute disseminated encephalomyelitis in children and adults: A focused review emphasizing new developments. Mult Scler. 2021;27(8):1153-60.
13. Jarius S, Aktas O, Ayzenberg I, Berthele A, Giglhuber K, Häußler V, et al. Update on the diagnosis and treatment of neuromyelits optica spectrum disorders (NMOSD) - revised recommendations of the Neuromyelitis Optica Study Group (NEMOS). Part I: Diagnosis and differential diagnosis. J Neurol. 2023;270(7):3341-68.
14. Zara P, Dinoto A, Carta S, Floris V, Turilli D, Budhram A, et al. Non-demyelinating disorders mimicking and misdiagnosed as NMOSD: a literature review. Eur J Neurol. 2023;30(10):3367-76.
15. Kümpfel T, Giglhuber K, Aktas O, Ayzenberg I, Bellmann-Strobl J, Häußler V, et al. Update on the diagnosis and treatment of neuromyelitis optica spectrum disorders (NMOSD) - revised recommendations of the Neuromyelitis Optica Study Group (NEMOS). Part II: Attack therapy and long-term management [published correction appears in J Neurol. 2024;271(6):3702-7.
16. Bonnan M, Valentino R, Debeugny S, Merle H, Ferge JL, Mehdaoui H, et al. Short delay to initiate plasma exchange is the strongest predictor of outcome in severe attacks of NMO spectrum disorders. J Neurol Neurosurg Psychiatry. 2018;89:346-51.
17. Demuth S, Guillaume M, Bourre B, Ciron J, Zephir H, Sirejacob Y, et al.; NOMADMUS Study Group. Treatment regimens for neuromyelitis optica spectrum disorder attacks: a retrospective cohort study. J Neuroinflamm. 2022;19:62.
18. Jiao Y, Fryer JP, Lennon VA, Jenkins SM, Quek AM, Smith CY, et al. Updated estimate of AQP4-IgG serostatus and disability outcome in neuromyelitis optica. Neurology. 2013;81:1197-204.
19. Bruscolini A, Sacchetti M, La Cava M, Gharbiya M, Ralli M, Lambiase A, et al. Diagnosis and management of neuromyelitis optica spectrum disorders - An update. Autoimmun Rev. 2018;17(3):195-200.
20. Anderson M, Levy M. Advances in the long-term treatment of neuromyelitis optica spectrum disorder. J Cent Nerv Syst Dis. 2024;16: 11795735241231094.
21. Marignier R, Pittock SJ, Paul F, Kim HJ, Bennett JL, Weinshenker BG, et al. AQP4-IgG-seronegative patient outcomes in the N-MOmentum trial of inebilizumab in neuromyelitis optica spectrum disorder. Mult Scler Relat Disord. 2022;57:103356.
22. Yamamura T, Kleiter I, Fujihara K, Palace J, Greenberg B, Zakrzewska-Pniewska B, et al. Trial of Satralizumab in Neuromyelitis Optica Spectrum Disorder. N Engl J Med. 2019;381(22):2114-24.
23. Traboulsee A, Greenberg BM, Bennett JL, Szczechowski L, Fox E, Shkrobot S, et al. Safety and efficacy of satralizumab monotherapy in neuromyelitis optica spectrum disorder: a randomised, double-blind, multicentre, placebo-controlled phase 3 trial. Lancet Neurol. 2020;19(5): 402-12.
24. Zhang C, Zhang M, Qiu W, Ma H, Zhang X, Zhu Z, et al. Safety and efficacy of tocilizumab versus azathioprine in highly relapsing neuromyelitis optica spectrum disorder (TANGO): an open-label, multicentre, randomised, phase 2 trial. Lancet Neurol. 2020;19(5):391-401.
25. Yang S, Zhang C, Zhang TX, Feng B, Jia D, Han S, et al. A real-world study of interleukin-6 receptor blockade in patients with neuromyelitis optica spectrum disorder. J Neurol. 2023;270(1):348-56.
26. Mealy MA, Kim SH, Schmidt F, López R, Jimenez Arango JA, et al. Aquaporin-4 serostatus does not predict response to immunotherapy in neuromyelitis optica spectrum disorders. Mult Scler. 2018;24(13):1737-42.

CHAPTER 10

Vaccination Principles in Patients with Central Nervous System Demyelinating Disorders

Pritam Majumdar, Thomas Mathew

ABSTRACT

The disease-modifying therapies (DMTs) used for the treatment of central nervous system (CNS) demyelinating disorders alter immune functions, making patients more susceptible to certain infections, particularly those of viral origin. Vaccinations against these infections can help prevent them when patients are initiated and maintained on DMTs. Rituximab is a commonly used DMT in the management of demyelinating disorders such as multiple sclerosis (MS), neuromyelitis optica spectrum disorder (NMOSD), and myelin oligodendrocyte glycoprotein antibody-associated disease (MOGAD) in our country. In this chapter, we will describe different DMTs, commonly used in our country, infections that are predisposed by specific DMTs, and vaccines that may prevent these infections. We will also discuss the vaccinations recommended for various DMTs and their effect on immunological responses to vaccination. The timing and selection of patients for vaccination are crucial for ensuring an optimal vaccine response, and these aspects will be a key focus of our discussion. Additionally, we will review the recommendations for vaccinations in specific population groups who are particularly prone to infections, such as pregnant females, the elderly, and patients planning to travel to countries where certain infections are endemic.

Keywords: Vaccines, Multiple sclerosis, Neuromyelitis optica spectrum disorders (NMOSD), Myelin oligodendrocyte glycoprotein associated disorders (MOGAD), Disease modifying therapy (DMT), Infections and COVID-19.

INTRODUCTION

In our country, common central nervous system (CNS) demyelinating disorders include multiple sclerosis (MS), neuromyelitis optica spectrum disorder (NMOSD), and myelin oligodendrocyte glycoprotein antibody disorder (MOGAD). These diseases are of autoimmune origin.[1] The majority of patients with these disorders receive treatment with immunomodulatory and immunosuppressant drugs, rendering them vulnerable to various infections. Therefore, patients initiating these medications should receive vaccination against these infections that may arise due to the immunosuppressive effects of various therapeutic agents. However, vaccinations are known to potentially trigger relapses in these diseases, and immunosuppressive medications can also impact vaccine responses. This complex interplay is illustrated in **Figure 1**. In this chapter, we cover various aspects of vaccination in demyelinating disorders relevant to our country.

VACCINATION PRINCIPLES

Vaccination in MS patients depend on the type of disease-modifying therapy (DMT) being administered, as well as the patient's comorbid conditions and age. The commonly used DMTs are summarized in **Table 1.** The type of infections varies with the DMT administered, and these are summarized in **Table 2**. Based on the infections linked to each DMT, appropriate vaccines should be chosen. All killed/inactivated vaccines should be completed 4–6 weeks before, and live vaccines 4–8 weeks before, the initiation of DMTs. Live vaccines are contraindicated during DMT treatment.[2] Killed vaccines can be administered, but immunological

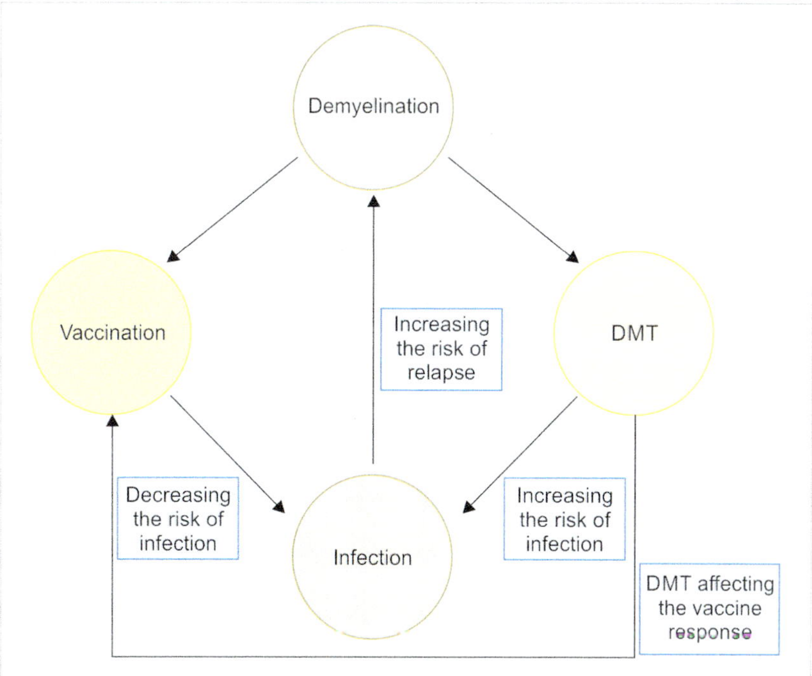

FIG. 1: The complex interplay between demyelination, disease-modifying therapy (DMT), infections, and vaccination.

TABLE 1: Commonly used DMTs in demyelinating disorders with increased risk of infections.[2]

Central demyelinating disorders	Commonly used DMTs
MS	Rituximab, natalizumab, ocrelizumab, alemtuzumab, IFN-β, dimethyl fumarate, fingolimod, glatiramer acetate, ofatumumab, and teriflunomide
NMOSD	Rituximab, azathioprine, glucocorticoids, mycophenolate mofetil, and eculizumab
MOGAD	Glucocorticoids, rituximab, azathioprine, mycophenolate mofetil, and tocilizumab

(DMT: disease-modifying therapy; IFN-β: Interferon-β; MS: multiple sclerosis; MOGAD: myelin oligodendrocyte glycoprotein antibody-associated disease; NMOSD: neuromyelitis optica spectrum disorder)

TABLE 2: Infections commonly associated with specific disease-modifying therapies.[2]

Immunomodulatory drugs	Associated infections	Vaccine-preventable infections
Anti CD20 therapy (rituximab, ocrelizumab, and ofatumumab)	JCV, HSV, VZV, HAV, HBV, HCV, and COVID-19	VZV, HAV, HBV, COVID-19
Natalizumab	JCV, HSV, VZV, COVID-19, and *Cryptococcus*	VZV, COVID-19
Alemtuzumab	HSV, VZV, HPV, HAV, HBV, HCV, CMV, COVID-19, *Candida*, TB, *Listeria*, and *Nocardia*	VZV, HPV, HAV, HBV, COVID-19
Teriflunomide	COVID-19	COVID-19
Dimethyl fumarate	JCV, COVID-19, *Cryptococcus*, and TB	COVID-19
Sphingosine-1 phosphate modulators (fingolimod, siponimod, and ozanimod)	JCV, HSV, VZV, HPV, COVID-19, *Cryptococcus*, and TB	HPV, VZV, COVID-19
Anti-IL-6 therapies (satralizumab, tocilizumab)	COVID-19	COVID-19
Anti-C5 inhibitor (eculizumab)	COVID-19, *Neisseria meningitidis*, *Haemophilus influenzae*	COVID-19, *Neisseria meningitidis*, *Haemophilus influenzae*

(JCV: John Cunningham virus; HSV: herpes simplex virus; VZV: varicella-zoster virus; HAV: hepatitis A virus; HBV: hepatitis B virus; HCV: hepatitis C virus; HPV: human papillomavirus; CMV: cytomegalovirus; COVID-19: Coronavirus disease 2019; TB: tuberculosis)

responses may vary with different DMTs, so measuring antibody titers is advised.[2] In the following sections, we will discuss vaccine recommendations for each commonly used DMT in detail.

RECOMMENDATIONS FOR VACCINATION WITH SPECIFIC DISEASE-MODIFYING THERAPIES[2,3]

Common Screening and Vaccinations for All Disease-modifying Therapies[2]

- *Mandatory infections to be ruled out at screening:*
    - Hepatitis B virus (HBV)
    - Hepatitis C virus (HCV)
    - Human immunodeficiency virus (HIV)
    - Tuberculosis (TB)
    - Syphilis
    - Varicella zoster virus (VZV) serology

Important: Rule out latent HBV infection by testing for Anti-HBcAb (core antibody).

- *Recommended vaccinations:*
    - Pneumococcal
    - Annual influenza [optional and as per the latest World Health Organization (WHO) recommendations for the southern hemisphere]
    - VZV (if seronegative)
    - HBV (optional and if seronegative):
        - If Anti-HBcAb is positive (must), vaccination should be done in consultation with gastroenterology under antiviral cover.

Rituximab

Rituximab is a commonly prescribed DMT for CNS demyelinating disorders. Before initiating rituximab, one should follow standard protocols and recommendations.

- *Screening*: Same as mentioned in screening for common infections and vaccination for all DMTs.
- *Recommended vaccinations*: Same as mentioned in screening for common infections and vaccination for all DMTs.
- *Interval between vaccine and medication:*
    - A minimum interval of 4 weeks is required between the last dose of a live or killed vaccine and the initiation of rituximab.
    - Live vaccines are not allowed during therapy.
    - Live vaccines can only be administered 12 months after the last dose of medication, and only if there is confirmed normal repopulation of B cells.

Ocrelizumab

- *Screening*: Same as mentioned in screening for common infections and vaccination for all DMTs.
- *Recommended vaccinations*: Same as mentioned in screening for common infections and vaccination for all DMTs.
- *Interval between vaccine and medication:*
    - A minimum interval of 6 weeks is required between the last dose of a live or killed vaccine and the initiation of DMT.
    - Live vaccines are not allowed during the therapy.
    - Live vaccines can only be administered after 18 months from the last dose of the medication, and only if there is a confirmed normal repopulation of B cells.

Ofatumumab

- *Screening*: Serum immunoglobulins need to be monitored. Rest same as mentioned in screening for common infections and vaccination for all DMTs.
- *Recommended vaccinations*: Same as mentioned in screening for common infections and vaccination for all DMTs.
- *Interval between vaccine and medication:*
    - A minimum interval of 6 weeks is required between the last dose of a live or killed vaccine and the initiation of ofatumumab.
    - Live vaccines are not allowed during the therapy.
    - Live vaccines can only be administered after 18 months from the last dose of the medication, and only if there is a confirmed normal repopulation of B cells.

Alemtuzumab

- *Screening*: Annual human papillomavirus (HPV) testing along with a pap smear examination should be done for females. Same as mentioned in screening for common infections and vaccination for all DMTs.
- *Recommended vaccinations*: Apart from the same vaccinations mentioned in screening for common infections and vaccination for all DMTs, it is also advised to consider HPV vaccination independently of age and sex.
- *Interval between vaccine and medication:*
    - A minimum interval of 6 weeks is required between the last dose of a live or killed vaccine and the initiation of alemtuzumab.
    - Live vaccines are not allowed while on the therapy.
    - Live vaccines can only be administered after 12 months from the last dose of the medication, and only if there is a confirmed normal repopulation of B cells.

Azathioprine

- *Screening*: Same as mentioned in screening for common infections and vaccination for all DMTs.
- *Recommended vaccinations*: Same as mentioned in screening for common infections and vaccination for all DMTs except regular Anti-HBcAb screening is not advised.
- *Interval between vaccine and medication*
    - For patients taking azathioprine, a minimum interval of 2–4 weeks is required between the last dose of a killed vaccine and the initiation of DMT, while a minimum interval of 4 weeks is required for live vaccines.
    - If a killed vaccine is administered at a much shorter interval, it is important to measure the vaccination responses.
    - Live vaccines are not allowed during the therapy and can only be administered 3 months after the last dose of the medication.

Cladribine

- *Screening*: Same as mentioned in screening for common infections and vaccination for all DMTs.
- *Recommended vaccinations*: Same as mentioned in screening for common infections and vaccination for all DMTs.
- *Interval between vaccine and medication:*
    - A minimum interval of 2–4 weeks is required between the last dose of a killed vaccine and the initiation of DMT, while a minimum interval of 4–6 weeks is required for live vaccines.
    - If a killed vaccine is administered at a much shorter interval, it is important to measure the vaccination responses.
    - Live vaccines are not allowed during the course of the therapy and can only be administered 3 months after the last dose of the medication.

Dimethyl Fumarate

- *Screening*: Same as mentioned in screening for common infections and vaccination for all DMTs, except regular Anti-HBcAb screening which is not advised.
- *Recommended vaccinations*: Same as mentioned in screening for common infections and vaccination for all DMTs.
- *Interval between vaccine and medication*
    - A minimum interval of 2–4 weeks is required between the last dose of a killed vaccine and the initiation of DMT, while a minimum interval of 4 weeks is required for live vaccines.
    - If a killed vaccine is administered at a much shorter interval, it is important to measure the vaccination responses.
    - Live vaccines are not allowed during the course of the therapy and can only be given when lymphocyte counts have normalized.

Fingolimod

- *Screening*: Known to cause VZV reactivation. Hence, VZV screening along with vaccination if antibody tests are negative. Also screen for other infections as mentioned in screening for common infections and vaccination for all DMTs.
- *Recommended vaccinations*: Same as mentioned in screening for common infections and vaccination for all DMTs.
- *Interval between vaccine and medication:*
    - A minimum interval of 2–4 weeks is required between the last dose of a killed vaccine and the initiation of DMT, while a minimum interval of 4 weeks is required for live vaccines.
    - If a killed vaccine is administered at a much shorter interval, it is important to measure the vaccination responses.
    - Live vaccines are not allowed during the course of the therapy and can only be administered 2 months after the last dose of the medication.

Glucocorticoids

No particular screening but exclude acute infection and avoid live vaccines. However, if an equivalent dose of 20 mg of prednisolone is planned for >2 weeks, then it is advisable to vaccinate with killed vaccines at least 2 weeks before and live vaccines at least 4 weeks before starting a patient on steroid therapy.

Natalizumab

- *Screening*: Same as mentioned in screening for common infections and vaccination for all DMTs.
- *Recommended vaccinations*: Same as mentioned in screening for common infections and vaccination for all DMTs.
- *Interval between vaccine and medication*
    - For patients planning this DMT, a minimum interval of 2–4 weeks is required between the last dose of a killed vaccine and the initiation of DMT, while a minimum interval of 4 weeks is required for live vaccines.
    - If a killed vaccine is administered at a much shorter interval, it is important to measure the vaccination responses.
    - Live vaccines are not allowed during the course of the therapy and can only be administered 2 months after the last dose of the medication.

Teriflunomide

- *Screening*: Apart from screening similar to common infections for all DMTs, it is also important to consider John Cunningham virus (JCV) screening to make therapeutic decisions.
- *Recommended vaccinations*: Same as mentioned in screening for common infections and vaccination for all DMTs.
- *Interval between vaccine and medication:*
    - A minimum interval of 2–4 weeks is required between the last dose of a killed vaccine and the initiation of DMT, while a minimum interval of 4 weeks is required for live vaccines.
    - If a killed vaccine is administered at a much shorter interval, it is important to measure the vaccination responses.
    - Live vaccines are not allowed during the course of the therapy and can only be administered 6 months after the last dose of the medication.

Tocilizumab

- *Screening*: Mandatory to exclude latent tuberculosis (TB) and HBV. The rest is the same as mentioned in screening for common infections and vaccination for all DMTs.
- *Recommended vaccinations*: Same as mentioned in screening for common infections and vaccination for all DMTs.
- *Interval between vaccine and medication:*
    - A minimum interval of 4 weeks is required between the last dose of a live or killed vaccine and the initiation of DMT.
    - Live vaccines are not allowed during the course of the therapy.

Mycophenolate Mofetil

Monitor complete blood count (CBC) and liver function test (LFT) in addition to the standard protocol for azathioprine.

Interferon beta

Annual influenza vaccination is recommended. Avoid live vaccines during the therapy. No interaction with vaccination responses.

Eculizumab

- *Screening*: Same as mentioned in screening for common infections and vaccination for all DMTs.

TABLE 3: Various types of vaccination.[5]

Types	Description	Advantages	Disadvantages	Examples
Live attenuated	Live virus weakened to keep them away from causing disease	Maximum immune response, 1–2 doses can provide lifetime protection	Chance of reactivation, requirement of cold chain	Measles, mumps, rubella, yellow fever, influenza, oral polio, typhoid, Japanese encephalitis, rotavirus, BCG, varicella zoster
Messenger RNA vaccines (mRNA)	Viral proteins given as antigens	Short manufacturing time, no live virus	Low immunogenicity	COVID-19
Subunit vaccines (polysaccharide, purified protein, recombinant protein, and peptide)	Constituent particles of the microorganism—such as its protein, sugar, or capsid	Excellent immune responses	Booster doses required	Pertussis, influenza, hepatitis B, meningococcal pneumococcal, typhoid, hepatitis A
Toxoid vaccines	Toxin made by the germ causing the disease	Specific, no live virus	Booster doses required	Diphtheria, tetanus
Virus vector vaccines	Modified product of virus to deliver antigen	Increases the immunogenicity, can be transported without a cold chain	Preexisting immunity against adenovirus can lead to decreased efficacy, injection site, and allergic reactions	Ebola, COVID-19
Killed vaccines	Killed or inactivated microorganisms	Safe, does not require cold chain	Weakly immunogenic, multiple doses and adjuvant required	Whole-cell pertussis, polio, influenza, Japanese encephalitis, hepatitis A, rabies

(BCG: Bacillus Calmette–Guérin; COVID-19: coronavirus disease of 2019; RNA: ribonucleic acid)

- *Recommended vaccinations*: The meningococcal vaccine (covering serogroups A, C, Y, W-135, and B) for all age groups along with *Haemophilus influenzae* and pneumococcal vaccines if the patient is under 18 years old, are required in addition to the vaccination protocol as followed for common vaccinations for all DMTs.
- *Interval between vaccine and medication:*
    - A minimum interval of 4 weeks is required between the last dose of a live or killed vaccine and the initiation of DMT.
    - Live vaccines are not allowed during the course of the therapy **(Table 3)**.

Figure 2 shows normal immunological response to vaccination.[4]

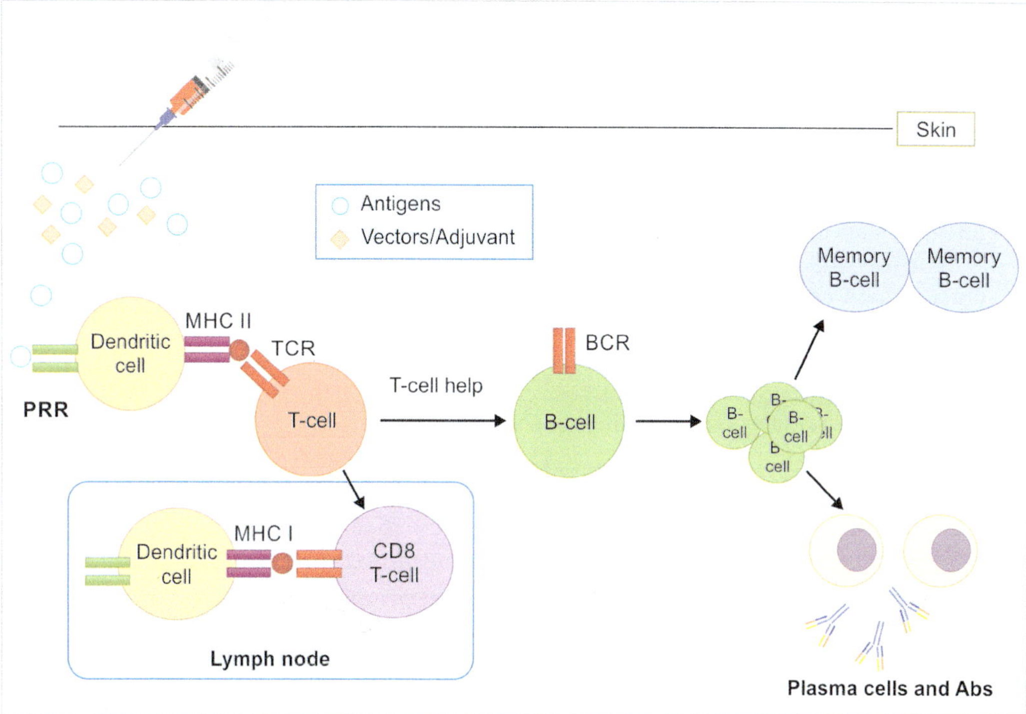

FIG. 2: Normal vaccination response—When a vaccination antigen is introduced, it is recognized by pattern recognition receptors (PRRs) on dendritic cells. These dendritic cells then present the antigen to T cells via T-cell receptor (TCR) using major histocompatibility complex (MHC) class II molecules. This interaction helps via B-cell receptor (BCR) B cells in the lymph nodes to develop and mature into antibody-producing plasma cells, which cause an initial surge of antibodies approximately 2 weeks postvaccination. B cells also mature into memory B cells, which migrate to bone marrow niches to continuously produce antibodies over a long period. Additionally, T cell help is required for CD8 T cells to differentiate into effector and memory CD8 T cells, contributing to long-term immunity and rapid response upon re-exposure to the antigen.

SPECIFIC VACCINES AND THEIR ADMINISTRATION[2,6]

Killed/Inactivated Vaccines

- *Herpes zoster virus:* Available as an inactivated (recombinant) vaccine (Shingrix), administered as two intramuscular (IM) doses separated by 2–6 months. It is recommended for patients aged over 18 years who are being treated with cladribine, alemtuzumab, sphingosine-1-phosphate (S1P) modulators, natalizumab, and anti-CD20 drugs. However, it is important to note that live vaccines are also available and should be avoided in these patients.
- *Seasonal influenza:* The influenza vaccine is available as inactivated fractions or subunits and is administered as a single IM or subcutaneous (SC) dose annually. The composition of the vaccine changes each year based on guidelines released by the WHO for the southern hemisphere in September.

For 2024, the WHO has recommended the following strains for the trivalent influenza vaccine:

- A/Victoria/4897/2022 (H1N1)pdm09-like virus
- A/Thailand/8/2022 (H3N2)-like virus
- B/Austria/1359417/2021 (B/Victoria lineage)-like virus

  For the quadrivalent influenza vaccines, which can be egg or cell culture-based or recombinant, the WHO also recommended the inclusion of the B/Yamagata lineage component—B/Phuket/3073/2013 (B/Yamagata lineage)-like virus.

  The influenza vaccine is particularly recommended for individuals considering immunotherapies and/or those with significant disabilities. Special considerations include administration during any trimester of pregnancy, especially in the context of present or future immunosuppression (IS).
- *Pneumococcal:* Available as an inactivated vaccine, pneumococcal conjugate vaccine (PCV13) followed by pneumococcal polysaccharide vaccine (PPSV23) with at least a 2-month interval between the two is recommended annually, especially if the patient is being considered for future immunotherapy and/or has significant disability. A booster dose with PPV23 is recommended after 5 years if needed.
- *Tetanus diphtheria (dT) or diphtheria pertussis tetanus (dTap):* Available as an inactivated vaccine. It should be administered as three IM doses (at 0, 1, and 6 months) in naïve patients. A single IM booster dose should be given to those previously vaccinated. The same schedule should be followed as for the general population. It is important to administer this vaccine during pregnancy, between the second and third trimesters, and to repeat it during each subsequent pregnancy.
- *Human papillomavirus:* Available as inactivated (recombinant) vaccine, given as three IM doses at months 0, 2, and 6. Consider in women and men with MS who will receive treatment with alemtuzumab independently of their age.
- *Hepatitis B vaccine:* Available as an inactivated (recombinant) vaccine and administered as regular vaccines in three IM doses at months 0, 1, and 6.

Consider this vaccination for high-risk populations such as those with a risk of sexual exposure, patients on dialysis, parenteral drug users, healthcare workers with occupational risk, and patients with specific comorbidities (HIV or HCV infection, chronic liver or kidney disease, solid organ transplant/hematopoietic stem cell transplantation recipients, and/or people receiving blood products), especially if treatment with anti-CD20 drugs is being considered.

Live-attenuated Vaccines

Live vaccines should always be avoided in MS patients already receiving the following immunosuppressive therapies: S1P modulators, anti-CD20 monoclonal antibodies, natalizumab, dimethyl fumarate (DMF), teriflunomide, and before immune restoration for cladribine and alemtuzumab.

In very exceptional cases, such as where there is a high risk of infection, vaccination with live-attenuated vaccines could be considered if the potential risk of acquiring the infection is superior to the risk of development of vaccine-related infections.

- *Measles, mumps, and rubella (MMR):* Available as a live-attenuated vaccine, administered as two IM or SC doses given 4 weeks apart. The vaccination must be completed at least 4 weeks before starting IS, as it is a live vaccine.
- *Varicella zoster virus:* Available as a live-attenuated vaccine, administered as two IM or SC doses given 4 weeks apart.

It is generally recommended for VZV seronegative patients. The vaccination must be completed at least 4 weeks before starting IS, as it is a live vaccine.

EFFECT OF DISEASE-MODIFYING THERAPIES ON VACCINE-RELATED IMMUNOLOGICAL RESPONSES

Disease-modifying drugs in MS can impact the immune response to vaccinations, necessitating careful timing and selection of vaccines to ensure effective immunization and minimize disease relapse or progression. Let us examine how each DMT affects the vaccine response and analyze the available evidence for each one **(Table 4)**.

CORONAVIRUS DISEASE OF 2019 AND VACCINATION IN PEOPLE WITH MULTIPLE SCLEROSIS

Risk of Coronavirus Disease of 2019 in People with Multiple Sclerosis

The risk of increased incidence of coronavirus disease of 2019 (COVID-19) in people with multiple sclerosis (PwMS) has not been established in studies.[27] However, PwMS on immunotherapy, particularly those receiving sphingosine-1 receptor blockers, cladribine, B-cell therapy, and alemtuzumab, have demonstrated increased severity of COVID-19, as reported in numerous studies.[28] Additionally, findings from our study indicate an increased hospitalization rate in these patients **(Table 5)**.[29]

Coronavirus Disease Vaccine Responses in Multiple Sclerosis Patients on Immunotherapy

Overall, B-cell depleting therapies and sphingosine-1 receptor blockers (fingolimod and siponimod) have been found to attenuate the response to the COVID-19 vaccine.[31] A study comparing the BNT162b2 vaccine antibody responses among 98 MS patients receiving cladribine, fingolimod, ocrelizumab, or no treatment found that responses in the cladribine and no-treatment groups were comparable and higher than those in the other two groups. The fingolimod group had the highest proportion of patients who did not develop adequate immune responses, while only 22% of the ocrelizumab group achieved adequate immune responses. However, there was no deterioration in disease course with any of the vaccines.[32] One interesting observation is that even if spike-specific and receptor-binding domain-specific antibodies remained low in patients with MS on B cell-depleting therapies, the antigen-specific T-cell response was comparable to that of healthy controls.[33] The only long-term follow-up study of 6 months reported protective antibody titers in 9.5% of patients in the fingolimod group, 22.8% in the ocrelizumab group, and 86% in the alemtuzumab group.[34]

Recommendations

It is because of this decrease in humoral response in patients receiving B-cell depleting therapy, fingolimod, and alemtuzumab, it is recommended to vaccinate at least 3 months after the last dose and 6–8 weeks before the next dose.[35]

RECOMMENDATIONS IN SPECIAL SITUATIONS

Pregnancy

Pregnant patients are considered a high-risk group for vaccine-preventable infectious diseases. The vaccination recommendations for pregnant patients with MS align with those for the general pregnant population. Notably, influenza and pertussis vaccines are

TABLE 4: Effect of disease-modifying therapies vaccine-related immunological responses.

DMT	Evidence	Inferences	Recommendations
Rituximab	• Kim et al., in a study including 26 patients with NMOSD, nine patients with multiple sclerosis (MS), and eight healthy controls found that patients on rituximab had the lowest geometric mean titers and seroprotection rates compared to those on azathioprine, interferon-beta (IFN-β), and healthy controls when tested at 3 and 5 weeks after influenza vaccination[7] • Vaccine trials in patients with rheumatoid arthritis (RA) compared the vaccination response to tetanus, keyhole limpet hemocyanin (KLH), and 23-valent pneumococcal polysaccharide vaccine (PPSV23), as well as delayed-type hypersensitivity to *Candida albicans* at 4 weeks, between patients receiving rituximab with methotrexate and those receiving only methotrexate. The results showed a comparable response to the tetanus vaccine and *Candida albicans* in both groups. However, the response to KLH and PPSV23 was decreased among patients receiving rituximab with methotrexate[8]	Immune responses following rituximab are impaired	It is recommended to vaccinate patients 4 weeks before administering rituximab. This can be applied to other B cell-depleting therapies in which evidence is lacking, such as oftamumab and inebilizumab
Ocrelizumab (OCR)	Amit et al.[9] examined the response to vaccination in 68 patients with relapsing-remitting multiple sclerosis (RRMS) undergoing treatment with ocrelizumab and 34 controls. Their study demonstrated a decreased response to the tetanus toxoid (TT)-containing vaccine after 8 weeks, and to pneumovax [23-valent (23-PPSV)] and KLH after 4 weeks in the ocrelizumab group. The primary ocrelizumab group was then randomized into two subgroups. OCR1 received Prevnar (13-valent conjugate pneumococcal vaccine) 4 weeks after 23-PPSV, while the OCR2 and control groups received the influenza vaccine. Prevnar did not seem to enhance the response to 23-PPSV in the OCR1 group, and a decreased response to the influenza vaccine was observed in the OCR2 group compared to controls. Despite the decreased responses, patients on ocrelizumab still mounted protective responses, which is why seasonal influenza vaccines are still recommended for patients on this treatment	No clear inference. Further trials needed	However, to achieve an optimal response, it is better to vaccinate patients 4 weeks before the start of therapy

Continued

Continued

DMT	Evidence	Inferences	Recommendations
Alemtuzumab	In the study conducted by McCarthy et al.,[10] serum antibody responses and seroconversion rates were found to be normal for T cell-dependent recall antigens (tetanus, diphtheria, and polio), a T cell-dependent novel antigen (meningococcus C), and T cell-independent antigens (pneumococcal), even at a follow-up of 6 months. However, the study did not include control groups and instead compared the responses with available data from normal patients, which raises concerns about the validity of the comparisons	No clear inference. Further trials needed	It is recommended to vaccinate patients 4 weeks before starting alemtuzumab therapy
Teriflunomide	• In 2011–2012, a study examined postvaccination antibody titers to seasonal influenza (H1N1, H3N2, and B groups) in patients with MS undergoing treatment with 7 or 14 mg of teriflunomide and IFN-β. The study found that the responses were normal for all vaccine groups except for a lesser response to the H1N1 vaccine among patients taking 14 mg of teriflunomide. The seroconversion rate was also lower in this group[11] • A randomized double-blind, placebo-controlled trial measured the response to rabies vaccination in patients with MS on teriflunomide compared to healthy controls. The study found a lesser response in the MS patients on teriflunomide; however, all patients achieved satisfactory seroconversion Additionally, the delayed-type hypersensitivity response to *Candida albicans*, Trichophyton, and tuberculin (recall antigens) was similar between the two groups[12]	There is no significant difference in vaccination responses among patients treated with teriflunomide compared to healthy controls	A variable response in one of the aforementioned trials with a 14 mg dose led to recommendations that vaccinations be completed at least 4 weeks before the start of treatment
Azathioprine	There was no decrease in response either to influenza vaccination nor to the preexisting antibodies of hepatitis B, measles, or rubella in a small group of patients receiving azathioprine for any neuroimmunological disease[7]	No difference in response as compared to healthy controls	Can be vaccinated anytime during therapy
Mycophenolate mofetil (MMF)	A study conducted on patients with NMO showed decreased antibody responses and seroconversion rates to influenza vaccines in those taking MMF compared to patients on azathioprine and IFN-β[7]	Immune responses following MMF are impaired	It is recommended to administer either booster doses of vaccinations or doses adjusted according to antibody titers measured over a period of time

Continued

Continued

DMT	Evidence	Inferences	Recommendations
Natalizumab	Two randomized controlled trials (RCTs) have confirmed that patients on natalizumab mount similar responses to vaccinations as healthy controls: • One study involved 17 patients receiving natalizumab and compared their antibody titers to the trivalent influenza A/B vaccine with those of 10 healthy controls. At the end of 12 weeks, the antibody were similar between the two groups, and interestingly, the titers were higher in the natalizumab group at the end of 4 weeks[13] • In another randomized open-label trial, an adequate response, defined by a ≥2-fold increase in antibody titers to tetanus toxoid and KLH, was achieved by a similar number of MS patients who were natalizumab-naive and those who had been on natalizumab treatment for 6 months[14]	No difference in response as compared to healthy controls	It is recommended to vaccinate at least 4 weeks before natalizumab, if it is not urgent
Fingolimod	• In a randomized, blinded, multicenter study, patients with MS receiving fingolimod had a lower response to seasonal influenza and tetanus booster vaccinations compared to healthy controls[15] • In another study where 11 MS patients received an attenuated live vaccine for VZV just before starting fingolimod. It was observed that seroconversion was achieved when fingolimod was started 26–27 days after the second dose of the vaccine. However, retesting at a median period of 2.42 years showed a global reduction in antibody titers in the fingolimod group[16]	Fingolimod significantly affects vaccination response	Vaccinate 4 weeks before starting fingolimod and check antibody levels regularly after the start of therapy. Give booster doses if levels go below subtherapeutic levels
Dimethyl fumarate (DMF)	In a single-center open-label study, the response to different vaccines was compared in 38 patients with MS receiving DMF and those receiving nonpegylatedIFNs. The vaccines tested were: • *Tetanus-diphtheria toxoid*: To assess T cell-dependent recall response • *Pneumococcal 23*: A polyvalent vaccine to evaluate T cell-independent humoral response • *Meningococcal oligosaccharide CRM197 conjugate vaccine (groups A, C, W-135, and Y)*: To test T cell-dependent neoantigen response[17]	No significant effect on vaccination response	It is recommended to vaccinate at least 4 weeks before natalizumab, if it is not urgent. If required can be given after start of therapy

Continued

Continued

DMT	Evidence	Inferences	Recommendations
Tocilizumab	• Evidence largely supports that tocilizumab does not significantly blunt immune responses to vaccinations. For example, one study demonstrated a higher seroconversion rate for the hepatitis B vaccine with tocilizumab compared to rituximab[18] • Additionally, trials involving RA patients showed no diminished response to influenza and PPSV when treated with tocilizumab[19] • However, a trial involving 112 patients with various autoimmune diseases found lower responses to pneumococcal conjugate vaccine (PCV13) and PPSV23 vaccines with tocilizumab[20]	While the evidence is somewhat mixed, the majority of studies suggest that tocilizumab does not significantly reduce vaccine responses	It is recommended to vaccinate at least 4 weeks before natalizumab if it is not urgent. If required can be given after the start of therapy
Glucocorticoids (GC)	• Glucocorticoids given at low doses ≤20 mg do not affect vaccination responses as seen in studies[21,22] • However, at high doses, there seems to be a concern as shown in studies. In one study of patients with RA receiving prednisolone >7.5 mg, the response was attenuated to PPSV and conjugate vaccine[20] • This attenuated response was also seen in another study with SLE patients receiving >20 mg of corticosteroids[23]	At high doses (>20 mg predniso-lone) can affect immune responses	It is recommended to monitor the titers and give booster vaccine accor-ding to them in patients receiving >20 mg of prednisolone or bioequivalent doses of other steroids
IVIg and plasmapheresis	We lack trials specifically addressing vaccine responses during plasma exchange or IVIg therapy. However, these therapies can neutralize the antigen if vaccines are administered within 4 weeks of treatment. Plasma exchange can also remove antibodies along with the exchange process	Immune responses are generally well established, 1–2 weeks after therapy	It is not recommended to administer any vaccines within 2–4 weeks before or during plasma exchange or IVIg. Wait for 1–2 weeks after the end of the procedure[24]

Continued

Continued

DMT	Evidence	Inferences	Recommendations
Stem cell transplantation	Vaccination is recommended according to stem cell implantation guidelines, which advise vaccinations against pneumococcus, tetanus, diphtheria, pertussis, poliomyelitis, *Haemophilus influenzae*, and annual influenza[25,26]		All vaccinations should be administered 3–6 months after transplantation to allow for immune reconstitution. Live-attenuated vaccines, such as those for measles, mumps, rubella, or VZV, are recommended only for patients in whom antibodies are not detectable after complete immune reconstitution

(IVIg: intravenous immunoglobulin; NMO: neuromyelitis optica; NMOSD: neuromyelitis optica spectrum disorder; RA: rheumatoid arthritis; SLE: systemic lupus erythematosus; VZV: varicella zoster virus)

TABLE 5: Various types of coronavirus disease of 2019 vaccines worldwide.[30]

Types	Specifications	Carrier	Name of vaccinations	First authorized	Adverse events
mRNA vaccines	Self-replicating RNA or mRNA (behave as killed vaccines)	Lipid nanoparticles	Pfizer BioNTech and Moderna	Germany, US	Severe anaphylaxis with Pfizer BioNTech
Nonreplicating adenovirus vector vaccines	Coronavirus DNA	Adenovirus	• Oxford–AstraZeneca • Sputnik V • Convidecia • Janssen • Covishield	US, Sweden Russia China US Netherlands India	NA
Inactivated vaccines	Formaldehyde killed culture grown virus		• CoronaVac • Sinopharm BIBP • WIBP vaccines • Covaxine • CoviVac • QazVac • COVIran Bareka	China China China India Russia Kazakhstan Iran	NA
Subunit vaccines	Protein fragments		• EpiVacCorona • MVC-COV1901 • Corbevax • Sanofi–GSK • Soberana 02	Russia Taiwan India, US France, UK Cuba	NA

(DNA: deoxyribonucleic acid; mRNA: messenger ribonucleic acid; NA: not available) particularly recommended for this group.[36,37] Vaccination with dTap vaccine during midpregnancy, around 20–36 weeks, provides both active and passive antibodies to the neonates, offering protection in the postnatal period. However, influenza vaccines can be given anytime.[38,39] The consensus in European guidelines is that killed vaccines can be administered at any time during pregnancy, though they should ideally be completed 2 weeks before administering any DMT. Live vaccines are not recommended at any time during pregnancy due to the risk of perinatal infection.[38] They can be given in the postnatal period even during breastfeeding (except yellow fever vaccines), and at least 4–6 weeks before starting any DMT.[2]

International Travel

For patients on immunotherapy, it is recommended to consult an MS/travel/infectious disease specialist 2–3 months before the date of departure. Killed vaccines such as hepatitis A, hepatitis B, rabies, Japanese encephalitis, quadrivalent meningococcal vaccine, cholera vaccine, tick-borne encephalitis (TBE), polio [inactivated poliovirus vaccine (IPV)], and inactivated typhoid vaccine have no contraindications. Conversely, live-attenuated vaccines against yellow fever, oral typhoid, dengue, varicella, and/or MMR are not recommended. Additionally, it is advised to check antibody titers for vaccines with standardized cutoffs to assess the need for repeat vaccination.[2]

Elderly

Immunosenescence in the elderly is known to reduce the efficacy of all vaccines in producing a response.[40,41] However, some vaccines have been specifically indicated for this age group, including the recombinant subunit herpes zoster virus vaccine, the pneumococcal vaccines, the adjuvanted or high-dose influenza vaccines, and booster vaccinations against tetanus and diphtheria. The European consensus recommends the same vaccination schedule as for a young adult, with additional consideration given to these vaccines specifically suited for older adults.[2]

KEY POINTS

- All killed/inactive vaccinations should be completed 4–6 weeks before, and live vaccinations 4–8 weeks before, the initiation of DMTs.
- Live vaccines are contraindicated during treatment with DMTs.
- Killed vaccines can be administered, but immunological responses to them can be variable with different DMTs, so a quantitative measure with antibody titers is advised.
- DMTs such as natalizumab and DMF have a minimal effect on vaccine responses and can be considered in patients who require both vaccination and urgent treatment.
- COVID-19 vaccinations should be administered 6–8 weeks before starting any DMTs.
- Influenza and pertussis vaccinations are highly recommended during pregnancy.
- Before traveling outside the country, a consultation with an MS expert is needed 2–3 months in advance to plan vaccinations.

CONCLUSION

The immunosuppressive DMTs used to treat CNS demyelinating disorders may predispose patients to certain infections, especially viral ones. Therefore, it is preferable to vaccinate these patients according to local guidelines and standard protocols. Except for live vaccines, all other killed vaccines appear to be safe for this group of patients. The decision on whom to vaccinate depends mainly on the type of DMT, baseline immune status, risk of infections, and special situations such as pregnancy, advanced age, or plans to travel to regions where certain diseases are endemic. After deciding whom to vaccinate, it is also important to determine the appropriate time for vaccination to ensure it produces an optimal response without interfering with the natural course of the disease. Our chapter addresses most of these questions to guide physicians and neurologists regarding vaccinations in CNS demyelinating disorders.

Declaration of generative AI and AI-assisted technologies in the writing process: During the preparation of this work the author(s) used ChatGPT (3.5) to refine language and grammar as a writing tool. After using this tool/service, the author(s) reviewed and edited the content as needed and take(s) full responsibility for the content of the publication.

REFERENCES

1. Lopez JA, Denkova M, Ramanathan S, Dale RC, Brilot F. Pathogenesis of autoimmune demyelination: from multiple sclerosis to neuromyelitis optica spectrum disorders and myelin oligodendrocyte glycoprotein antibody-associated disease. Clin Transl Immunology. 2021;10(7):e1316.
2. Tur C, Dubessy AL, Otero-Romero S, Amato MP, Derfuss T, Di Pauli F, et al. The risk of infections for multiple sclerosis and neuromyelitis optica spectrum disorder disease-modifying treatments: Eighth European Committee for Treatment and Research in Multiple Sclerosis Focused Workshop Review. April 2021. Mult Scler. 2022;28(9):1424-56.
3. Winkelmann A, Loebermann M, Barnett M, Hartung HP, Zettl UK. Vaccination and immunotherapies in neuroimmunological diseases. Nat Rev Neurol. 2022;18(5):289-306.
4. Pollard AJ, Bijker EM. A guide to vaccinology: from basic principles to new developments. Nat Rev Immunol. 2021;21(2):129.
5. HHS government. (2022). Vaccine types. [online] Available from https://www.hhs.gov/immunization/basics/types/index.html. [Last accessed September, 2024].
6. World Health Organization. (2024). Recommended composition of influenza virus vaccines for use in the 2024 southern hemisphere influenza season. [online] Available from https://www.who.int/publications/m/item/recommended-composition-of-influenza-virus-vaccines-for-use-in-the-2024-southern-hemisphere-influenza-season. [Last accessed September, 2024].
7. Kim W, Kim SH, Huh SY, Kong SY, Choi YJ, Cheong HJ, et al. Reduced antibody formation after influenza vaccination in patients with neuromyelitis optica spectrum disorder treated with rituximab. Eur J Neurol. 2013;20(6):975-80.
8. Bingham CO 3rd, Looney RJ, Deodhar A, Halsey N, Greenwald M, Codding C, et al. Immunization responses in rheumatoid arthritis patients treated with rituximab: results from a controlled clinical trial. Arthritis Rheum. 2010;62(1):64-74.
9. Bar-Or A, Calkwood JC, Chognot C, Evershed J, Fox EJ, Herman A, et al. Effect of ocrelizumab on vaccine responses in patients with multiple sclerosis: The VELOCE study. Neurology. 2020;95(14):e1999-e2008.
10. McCarthy CL, Tuohy O, Compston DA, Kumararatne DS, Coles AJ, Jones JL. Immune competence after alemtuzumab treatment of multiple sclerosis. Neurology. 2013;81(10):872-6.
11. Bar-Or A, Freedman MS, Kremenchutzky M, Menguy-Vacheron F, Bauer D, Jodl S, et al. Teriflunomide effect on immune response to influenza vaccine in patients with multiple sclerosis. Neurology. 2013;81(6):552-8.
12. Bar-Or A, Wiendl H, Miller B, Benamor M, Truffinet P, Church M, et al. Randomized study of teriflunomide effects on immune responses to neoantigen and recall antigens. Neurol Neuroimmunol Neuroinflamm. 2015;2(2):e70.
13. Vagberg M, Kumlin U, Svenningsson A. Humoral immune response to influenza vaccine in natalizumab- treated MS patients. Neurol Res. 2012;34:730-3.
14. Kaufman M, Pardo G, Rossman H, Sweetser MT, Forrestal F, Duda P. Natalizumab treatment shows no clinically meaningful effects on immunization responses in patients with relapsing-remitting multiple sclerosis. J. Neurol Sci. 2014;341(1-2):22-7.

15. Kappos L, Mehling M, Arroyo R, Izquierdo G, Selmaj K, Curovic-Perisic V, et al. Randomized trial of vaccination in fingolimod- treated patients with multiple sclerosis. Neurology. 2015;84(9):872-9.
16. Signoriello E, Bonavita S, Sinisi L, Russo CV, Maniscalco GT, Casertano S, et al. Is antibody titer useful to verify the immunization after VZV vaccine in MS patients treated with fingolimod? A case series. Mult Scler Relat Disord. 2020;40: 101963.
17. von Hehn C, Howard J, Liu S, Meka V, Pultz J, Mehta D, et al. Immune response to vaccines is maintained in patients treated with dimethyl fumarate. Neurol. Neuroimmunol Neuroinflamm. 2018;5:e409.
18. Richi P, Alonso O, Martín MD, González-Hombrado L, Navío T, Salido M, Llorente J, et al. Evaluation of the immune response to hepatitis B vaccine in patients on biological therapy: results of the RIER cohort study. Clin Rheumatol. 2020;39(9):2751-6.
19. Mori S, Ueki Y, Akeda Y, Hirakata N, Oribe M, Shiohira Y, et al. Pneumococcal polysaccharide vaccination in rheumatoid arthritis patients receiving tocilizumab therapy. Ann Rheum Dis. 2013;72:1362-6.
20. Richi P, Yuste J, Navío T, González-Hombrado L, Salido M, Thuissard-Vasallo I, et al. Impact of biological therapies on the immune response after pneumococcal vaccination in patients with autoimmune inflammatory diseases. Vaccines (Basel). 2021;9(3):203.
21. American Academy of Pediatrics. In: Pickering LK, Baker C, Kimberlin DW, Long S (Eds). Red Book: 2009 Report of the Committee on Infectious Diseases, 28th edition. Elk Grove Village, IL: American Academy of Pediatrics; 2009.
22. Bühler S, Eperon G, Ribi C, Kyburz D, van Gompel F, Visser LG, et al. Vaccination recommendations for adult patients with autoimmune inflammatory rheumatic diseases. Swiss Med Wkly. 2015;145: w14159.
23. Borba EF, Saad CG, Pasoto SG, Calich AL, Aikawa NE, Ribeiro AC, et al. Influenza A/H1N1 vaccination of patients with SLE: can antimalarial drugs restore diminished response under immunosuppressive therapy? Rheumatology. 2012;51:1061-9.
24. Guptill JT, Juel VC, Massey JM, Anderson AC, Chopra M, Yi JS, et al. Effect of therapeutic plasma exchange on immunoglobulins in myasthenia gravis. Autoimmunity. 2016;49(7):472-9.
25. Sharrack B, Saccardi R, Alexander T, Badoglio M, Burman J, Farge D, et al. Autologous haematopoietic stem cell transplantation and other cellular therapy in multiple sclerosis and immune-mediated neurological diseases: updated guidelines and recommendations from the EBMT Autoimmune Diseases Working Party (ADWP) and the Joint Accreditation Committee of EBMT and ISCT (JACIE). Bone Marrow Transpl. 2020;55(2): 283-306.
26. Christopeit M, Schmidt-Hieber M, Sprute R, Buchheidt D, Hentrich M, Karthaus M, et al. Prophylaxis, diagnosis and therapy of infections in patients undergoing high- dose chemotherapy and autologous haematopoietic stem cell transplantation. 2020 update of the recommendations of the Infectious Diseases Working Party (AGIHO) of the German Society of Hematology and Medical Oncology (DGHO). Ann Hematol. 2021;100(2):321-36.
27. Loonstra FC, Hoitsma E, van Kempen ZL, Killestein J, Mostert JP. COVID-19 in multiple sclerosis: the Dutch experience. Mult Scler. 2020;26(10): 1256-60.
28. Hartung HP, Aktas O. COVID-19 and management of neuroimmunological disorders. Nat Rev Neurol. 2020;16:347-8.
29. Mathew T, Garg S, John SK, Kimi MS, Chhakchhuak NZ, Koshy S, et al. COVID-19 Infection in Multiple Sclerosis Patients Treated with Rituximab Compared to Natalizumab and Healthy Controls: A Real-World Multicenter Study. Ann Indian Acad Neurol. 2024;27(3):264-8.
30. World Health Organization. (2024). The different types of COVID-19 vaccines. [online] Available from https://www.who.int/news-room/feature-stories/detail/the-race-for-a-covid-19-vaccine-explained. [Last accessed September, 2024].
31. Pawlitzki M, Zettl UK, Ruck T, Rolfes L, Hartung HP, Meuth SG. Merits and culprits of immunotherapies for neurological diseases in times of COVID-19. EBioMedicine. 2020;56:102822.
32. Achiron A, Mandel M, Dreyer-Alster S, Harari G, Magalashvili D, Sonis P, et al. Humoral immune response to COVID-19 mRNA vaccine in patients with multiple sclerosis treated with high- efficacy disease- modifying therapies. Ther Adv Neurol Disord. 2021;14:1-8.
33. Apostolidis SA, Kakara M, Painter MM, Goel RR, Mathew D, Lenzi K, et al. Cellular and humoral immune responses following SARS- CoV-2 mRNA vaccination in patients with multiple sclerosis on anti- CD20 therapy. Nat Med. 2021;27(11): 1990-2001.
34. Achiron A, Mandel M, Dreyer-Alster S, Harari G, Dolev M, Menascu S, et al. Humoral immune response in multiple sclerosis patients following PfizerBNT162b2 COVID19 vaccination: Up to

6 months cross-sectional study. J Neuroimmunol. 2021;361:577746.

35. Centonze D, Rocca MA, Gasperini C, Kappos L, Hartung HP, Magyari M, et al. Disease-modifying therapies and SARS-CoV-2 vaccination in multiple sclerosis: an expert consensus. J Neurol. 2021; 268(11):3961-8.
36. Cabreira V, Abreu P, Soares-Dos-Reis R, Guimarães J, Sá MJ. Multiple sclerosis, disease-modifying therapies and COVID-19: a systematic review on immune response and vaccination recommendations. Vaccines (Basel). 2021;9(7): 773.
37. Reyes S, Ramsay M, Ladhani S, Amirthalingam G, Singh N, Cores C, et al. Protecting people with multiple sclerosis through vaccination. Pract Neurol. 2020;20(6):435-45.
38. Swamy GK, Heine RP. Vaccinations for pregnant women. Obstet Gynecol. 2015;125(1):212-26.
39. Healy CM. Pertussis vaccination in pregnancy. Hum Vaccin Immunother. 2016;12(8):1972-81.
40. Cunningham AL, McIntyre P, Subbarao K, Booy R, Levin MJ. Vaccines for older adults. BMJ. 2021;372:n188.
41. Burke M, Rowe T. Vaccinations in older adults. Clin Geriatr Med. 2018;34(1):131-43.

CHAPTER

11

Pregnancy and Central Nervous System Demyelination

Kshiteeja Jain, Jayanth SS, Netravathi M

ABSTRACT

Central nervous system (CNS) demyelinating disorders comprise a heterogeneous group of immune-mediated disorders, each with its distinct pathogeneses. As most of them affect women predominantly, they often present in their childbearing years. Pregnancy is a unique immune-tolerant state and in turn influences the course of these neuroimmunological disorders. The outcomes differ significantly for each disorder, reflecting the impact of hormonal changes, immune subsets, and individual pathogenesis. Pregnancy is considered protective for multiple sclerosis (MS) with a decrease in relapse rate during pregnancy followed by a rebound increase in the immediate postpartum period. In contrast, several studies have suggested an increased relapse risk and higher disability during and immediately after pregnancy in aquaporin-4 positive neuromyelitis optica spectrum disorder (AQP4+ NMOSD) patients; however, a link between NMOSD and poor pregnancy outcomes such as miscarriage and preeclampsia have also been reported. Not enough is known about patients with myelin oligodendrocyte glycoprotein-associated disease (MOGAD) and dual-seronegative NMOSD and future studies are required to shed more light. It is our sincere effort to evaluate the available evidence in pregnancy and CNS demyelinating disorders and present a detailed review of the topic.

Keywords: Pregnancy, Breastfeeding, Central nervous system (CNS) demyelination, Multiple sclerosis (MS), Neuromyelitis optica spectrum disorder (NMOSD), Myelin oligodendrocyte glycoprotein-associated disease (MOGAD), Guidelines.

INTRODUCTION

Central nervous system (CNS) demyelinating disorders are a heterogeneous group of autoimmune disorders characterized by damage to the myelin sheath with relative sparing of the axons. They comprise multiple sclerosis (MS), neuromyelitis optica spectrum disorder (NMOSD), myelin oligodendrocyte glycoprotein-associated disease (MOGAD), and other secondary CNS demyelinating disorders. Most of these demyelinating disorders are more common in women and the initial clinical presentation for many is in the childbearing age group.

Pregnancy poses a unique challenge to the human immune system not because it broadly suppresses immunity but due to the distinct state of immune tolerance it creates. Pregnancy also influences the course of these neuroimmunological conditions. With each disorder, the outcomes of pregnancy would differ significantly, highlighting the impact of hormonal changes, T-cell subsets, and placental factors on disease pathogenesis.[1]

Historically, women with MS were advised to avoid pregnancy. However, recent evidence suggests that pregnancy does not negatively impact the progression of MS.[2] Over the last 20 years, there have been numerous studies, both retrospective and prospective, investigating this matter.[3,4] Previous studies have shown that around 90% of patients develop symptoms before the age of 50 years, and nearly one third among them become pregnant after they are diagnosed with MS. Hence, it is of paramount importance to consider discussing regarding marriage, family planning, and pregnancy with the patient while considering the treatment.[5] Over the last few decades, there has been a landmark development in the treatment of MS. Multiple disease-modifying treatments (DMTs) of variable efficacy have been developed which are also approved by the European Medicine Agency (EMA) and the United States Food and Drug Administration (FDA). Many DMTs are in the pipeline.

Compared to MS, available literature regarding NMOSD and pregnancy is scant, but it has been demonstrated that NMOSD and pregnancy can have reciprocal effects on each other.[6] Several studies have suggested an increased relapse risk and higher disability during and immediately after pregnancy,[7,8] whereas a link between NMOSD and poor pregnancy outcomes such as miscarriage and preeclampsia have also been reported.[9] Other autoimmune disorders frequently coexist with aquaporin-4 positive NMOSD (AQP4+ NMOSD) such as systemic lupus erythematosus (SLE), autoimmune thyroid diseases, coeliac disease, and/or myasthenia gravis in up to 25% patients and can affect pregnancy outcomes.[10]

MULTIPLE SCLEROSIS

Pregnancy and Immune System and its Effect on Multiple Sclerosis

The maternal-fetal interface consists of the placenta, which originates from the fetus, and the decidua, which is derived from the mother. Fetal cells interact directly with the maternal immune system through extravillous trophoblasts (EVTs). EVTs evade the maternal immune system and promote immune tolerance by expressing a distinctive set of major histocompatibility complex (MHC) molecules.[11] Human leukocyte antigen-G (HLA-G), a nonclassical MHC class 1 gene, which is highly expressed in trophoblasts, is shown to play a pivotal role in the immunological mechanisms that control maternal-fetal tolerance during pregnancy. It does so by inhibiting the cytotoxic activity of the natural killer cells and downregulating the T helper 1 (Th1) cytokine production.[12-14] It is also known that there is a transition from a Th1 to a T helper 2 (Th2) immune environment to maintain fetal tolerance **(Fig. 1)**.[15,16]

Pregnancy results in significant physiological changes in the body which is mainly influenced by the change in hormone levels including the sex hormones. Among them, the estrogen levels progressively increase throughout pregnancy, reaching 100 times the prenatal levels by the third trimester. Progesterone and 17 hydroxyprogesterone levels also grow steadily throughout the pregnancy.[17] Progesterone has been shown to stimulate the secretion of Th2 and reduce the secretion of Th1 cytokines which maintains pregnancy.[18] Human chorionic gonadotrophin (hCG) continues to rise during the first trimester, reaching its peak levels by the 12th week of gestation; the levels then fall rapidly during the second trimester to again slowly rise during the last trimester.

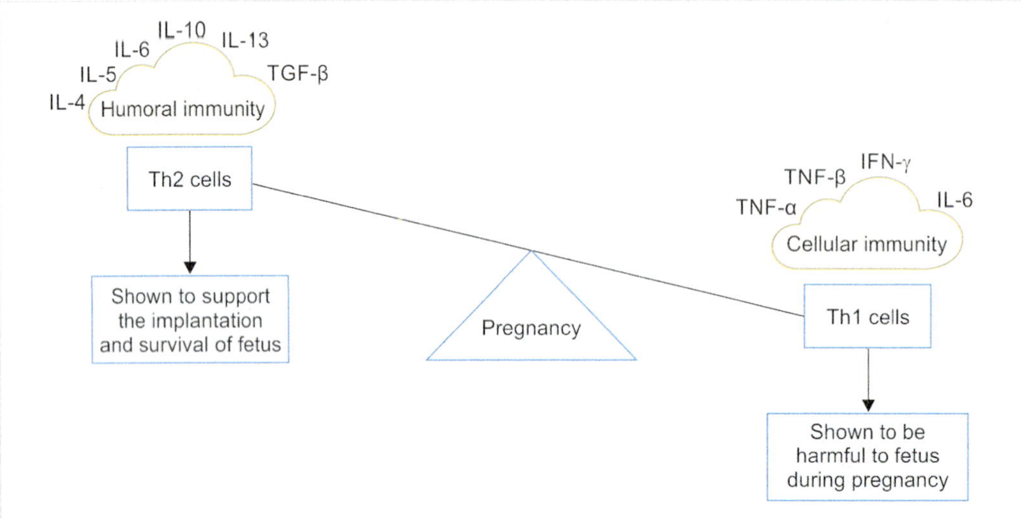

FIG. 1: Normal changes in immune molecules during pregnancy and its effect on the fetus and pregnancy. (IFN: interferon; IL: interleukin; TGF: transforming growth factor; Th1: T helper 1; Th2: T helper 2; TNF: tumor necrosis factor)

Multiple sclerosis is largely regarded as Th1-mediated disease.[19] Th1 cells play a pivotal role in the release of mediators which lead to an autoreactive inflammatory attack and myelin degeneration, which is one of the key processes involved in the pathogenesis of MS.[20] With the growing evidence and literature, it is well established that the relapse rate of MS tends to decrease during pregnancy, particularly in the third trimester but rises significantly after childbirth. As discussed earlier, there is an alteration in the repertoire of T cells from Th1 to Th2 during pregnancy. There will be increased production of Th2 cytokines, which inhibits the development of inflammatory Th1/Th17 cells.[21] Cytokines are secreted even from the fetoplacental unit which downregulates other cytokine-like substances mediating the mother's cellular immunity.[22] The relapse rates of MS during pregnancy are also influenced by these hormonal levels. There may be a relatively higher recurrence rate in the second trimester when compared to the first, due to the decrease in the hCG levels. However, the risk is significantly lower during the third trimester due to the peaking of the estrogen and progesterone levels.[23] The high recurrence rate in the postpartum period may be explained by the changing hormonal levels after pregnancy **(Flowchart 1)**.

Impact of Pregnancy on the Relapse Rate of Multiple Sclerosis

The first prospective study concerning the impact of pregnancy on MS was the Pregnancy in Multiple Sclerosis (PRIMS) study which included 254 patients with MS (269 pregnancies), where women were followed up during pregnancy and 2 years postpartum. The results showed that the rate of relapse of MS decreased throughout the pregnancy, mostly during the last trimester. However, there was an increase in the relapse rate 3 months after delivery which was similar to the prepregnancy relapse rates.[4] This observation was also made in a large retrospective study consisting of 2,158 successfully delivered patients with

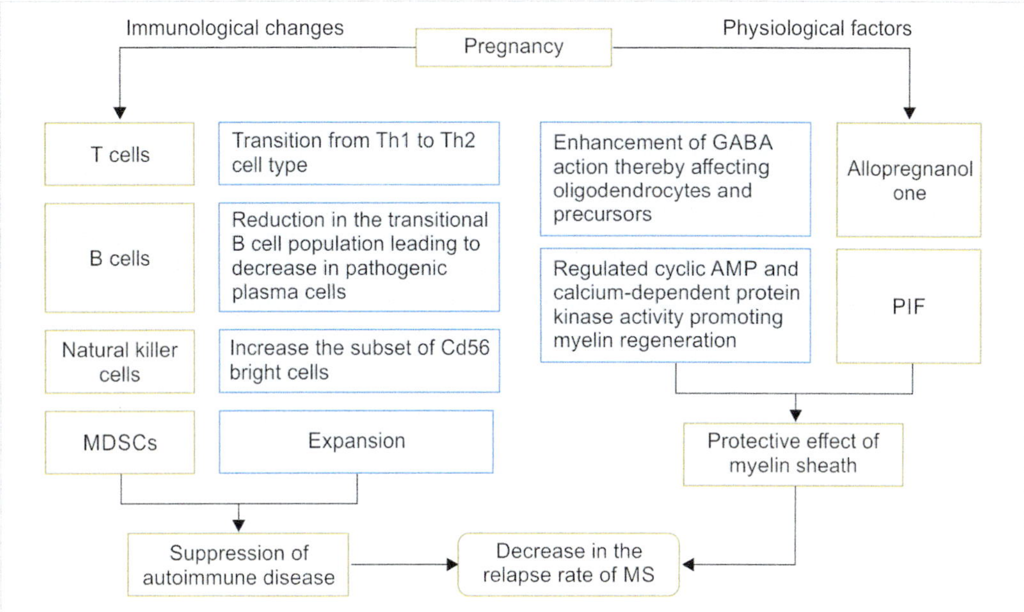

FLOWCHART 1: Mechanisms involved in the decrease in the relapse rate of MS during pregnancy.

(AMP: adenosine monophosphate; GABA: gamma-aminobutyric acid; MDSCs: myeloid-derived suppressor cells; MS: multiple sclerosis; PIF: preimplantation factor; Th1: T helper 1; Th2: T helper 2)

Source: Adapted from Wang Y, Wang J, Feng J. Multiple sclerosis and pregnancy: Pathogenesis, influencing factors, and treatment options. Autoimmun Rev. 2023;22(11):103449.

MS in the United States between 2006 and 2015.[24] These changes are due to the immunological changes during pregnancy and the physiological responses to myelin protection due to the fluctuating hormones during pregnancy.

Antepartum Planning

It is vital for clinicians to discuss the possibility and wishes for pregnancy with every MS patient of the childbearing age group. These discussions should happen as early as the patients are diagnosed with MS and never be delayed until the women with MS become pregnant. Patients with MS will also have concerns about fertility, the chances of transmitting MS to the child, the impact of DMTs and other drugs on pregnancy, pregnancy's influence on MS activity, and the capacity at which the mother can breastfeed and raise the child.[25] Before planning to conceive, a period of disease stability should be tried to achieve. However, this would be patient centric, with few requiring highly effective therapies while others requiring maintenance therapies. If there is a need to change the DMTs or a need for a washout period before planning for pregnancy, it should be carried out well in advance to minimize the risk of relapse and the possible exposure of the fetus to teratogens. If the patients are on symptomatic therapies, they should be advised regarding the safety and the potential risks associated with the medicine during pregnancy as well as breastfeeding. Care should be given to the mental health of the mother with intervention from the psychiatrist and the psychotherapists.

Effect on fertility: It has been observed throughout various studies that MS does not have any impact on fertility or the risk of miscarriage. These patients will also not carry any increased risk for premature or stillbirth, birth defects, cesarean delivery, or spontaneous abortions.[25] Patients with MS carry the same ability as healthy women to conceive.[26] This observation is observed in patients with stable disease or low expanded disability status scale (EDSS), but when the patients have features of myelopathy with significant urogenital issues, then the disability may pose a risk.

Is there a genetic risk? Pregnant women with MS will also have concerns of transmitting illness to the child. The risk of a child developing MS is 20–50 times higher than the general population if one of the parents has MS, although the absolute risk will only be 3–5%.[27] In the development of MS, genetic factors also play a prominent role with main attribution to the variants in genes that regulate the function of the immune system, such as HLADRB1*15:01 and FTO rs9939609.[28]

Contraception and family planning: Effective contraception is important for women with MS to avoid unwanted pregnancies. Use of oral contraceptives has been associated with an increased risk of worsening symptoms of MS, which is mainly due to the imbalance between the progesterone and the estrogen levels, leading to alteration of the maternal immune status.[29] Hence, the decision on the use and methods of contraception should be individualized according to the MS disease course, possible interactions with DMT in use, further treatment plans, and previous medical history. There are no restrictions on the use of intrauterine devices.[30]

Sexual dysfunction is a common symptom observed among patients with MS. A systematic review and meta-analysis conducted in 2018 showed that among 14,538 patients, 61% of men and 63% of women had problems with sexual intercourse. In the absence of sexual dysfunction, assistive reproductive technology (ART) will have to be considered in patients with MS.[31] However, these patients on ART who fail to conceive will have a higher risk of clinical or radiological worsening in the next 3 months and an increased annualized relapse rate (ARR).[32] The increased risk of relapses is linked to the usage of gonadotropin-releasing hormone (GnRH) agonists **(Flowchart 2)**.

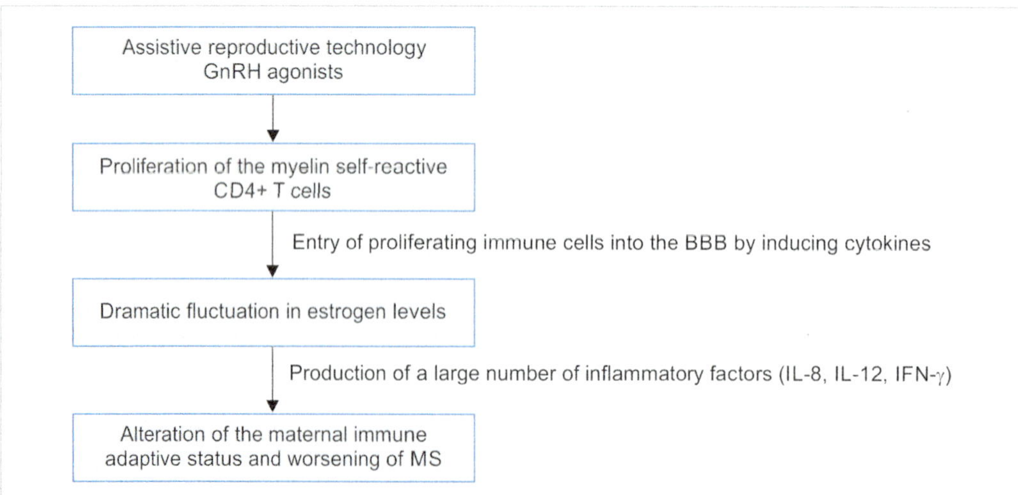

FLOWCHART 2: Mechanism behind the worsening of MS in patients on assistive reproductive technology.
(BBB: blood–brain barrier; GnRH: gonadotropin-releasing hormone; IFN: interferon; IL: interleukin; MS: multiple sclerosis)

However, continued use of DMT improved the relapse rate in patients with MS who are on ART.[33]

Along with the usage of folic acid and other vitamins, vitamin D supplementation is also recommended.

Multiple Sclerosis during Pregnancy

Multiple sclerosis team should be made aware of the pregnancy as soon as possible to provide adequate support and be in conjuncture with the obstetric team. During pregnancy, women with MS should be advised to abstain from alcohol and smoking and maintain a healthy diet. They should continue folic acid and vitamin D supplementations. MS is not known to affect the outcomes of pregnancy such as preeclampsia, chorioamnionitis, and postpartum hemorrhage.[34] Hence, pregnancy in MS need not be labeled as high risk. No additional obstetric scans are recommended for pregnant women with MS. Vaccination is an important aspect for patients on DMTs. In pregnant women with MS, specific modifications are required. Live vaccines have to be avoided during the pregnancy, whereas inactivated vaccines such as inactivated influenza and diphtheria can be given.[35-37] Magnetic resonance imaging (MRI) is considered to be safe during pregnancy with studies showing no increased risk of stillbirth, congenital malformations, tumors, or deafness in the fetus.[38] However, it has been observed that few sequences in the higher field strength (3 Tesla) can result in higher energy deposition to the fetus. Hence, MRI with low field strength is recommended.[39] Gadolinium contrast should be limited to situations where the risk is outweighed by the benefit, as it can cross the placental barrier and accumulate in the fetal brain, leading to adverse effects;[40] hence, it is better avoided.

There are a few conditions and comorbidities which are common during pregnancy in MS patients. Urinary tract infections (UTIs) are common during pregnancy. Patients should be made aware of the symptoms of UTI, helping them to recognize it early and seek the necessary advice.[41] A study of 171 pregnant women with MS showed that a reduction in the frequency of sexual intercourse and proper genital hygiene could aid in preventing infection.[42] Oral nitrofurantoin followed by amoxicillin and cefadroxil are recommended for UTI in pregnant women with MS. Intravenous antibiotics based on urine culture and sensitivity pattern are recommended in patients with pyelonephritis. Hypothyroidism is common during pregnancy and it is known to have an impact on the severity of MS in offspring, especially in patients on alemtuzumab.[43] This warrants a need for regular monitoring of the thyroid status.

Management of Relapses during Pregnancy

Some women with MS can have relapse during pregnancy, despite the reduction of disease activity. There are no contraindications for doing MRI during relapses, but gadolinium-enhanced contrast should be avoided. Intravenous methylprednisolone (IVMP) is the drug of choice during relapses in pregnancy. It can be administered after ruling out the underlying infection such as UTI. Previous studies have raised concerns about increased risk of oral clefts in the offspring when steroids are given in the first trimester, but recent studies have not observed these findings. Plasma exchange can be done in patients with severe relapse who are not responding to corticosteroids.

Disease-modifying Therapies during Pregnancy and Breastfeeding

Disease-modifying therapies during pregnancy must be tailored individually, considering the patient's views around the treatment during pregnancy, and the age, degree of disability, clinical and MRI disease activity, relapse rate, and the risk of continuing or terminating the treatment.[25]

Interferon-beta and Glatiramer Acetate

There is no available evidence from human studies indicating that interferon-beta (IFN-β) or glatiramer acetate (GA) affects the fertility of men or women or any risk of congenital malformations or miscarriage.[44] Both IFN-β and GA are sizable molecules and do not cross the placental barrier in any amount. They also do not interact with hormonal contraceptives.[45] None of the current evidence indicates a need for an abortion in case of an unplanned pregnancy with IFN-β and GA. Both IFN-β and GA may not be required in a few patients as the relapse rates fall during pregnancy. However, if the patient's condition warrants continuation, they can be continued as long as possible as there is no evidence indicating harm to the fetus.[44] If IFN-β and GA are stopped during pregnancy, they require time to reach their full efficacy once restarted and so the relapse rate might increase during the first few months after delivery.[44] Although there are reservations about the use of IFN-β during breastfeeding, both IFN-β and GA can be used during breastfeeding as the benefits outweigh the risks.[34]

Natalizumab

Natalizumab is an immunoglobulin G4 (IgG4) humanized monoclonal antibody (mAb) that acts against α4-integrin (cell adhesion molecule). It is not known to interact with hormonal contraception and there are no human studies suggesting reduced fertility or congenital malformations with natalizumab.[44]

With discontinuation of natalizumab, there is a risk of rebound and a sharp increase in the relapse rate, which usually occurs 12–16 weeks after stopping natalizumab.[46] Natalizumab will not enter the fetal circulation up to 13–14 weeks of gestation until the placenta is formed, but thereafter, it crosses the placenta during the second and third trimesters.[44,45] To minimize the exposure of the fetus to natalizumab, it is recommended to give the last dose at 34 weeks of pregnancy and reinitiate soon after the delivery, within 8–12 weeks after the last dose as much as to avoid rebound activity.[44] Although unlicensed, a study done on extended dosing intervals on natalizumab at 8-week intervals to reduce the exposure did not show any reduction in efficacy.[47] MRI brain imaging screening for progressive multifocal leukoencephalopathy can be continued during the pregnancy as required. Natalizumab is known to be secreted in breast milk and the amount increases with time.[48] However, the Association of British Neurologists MS Advisory Group panel recommends breastfeeding, as the oral bioavailability is negligible and any transfer into the breast milk is unlikely to result in systemic absorption by the baby.[44]

Fingolimod

Fingolimod, a sphingosine-1-phosphate inhibitor, was the first oral DMT approved for MS. Fingolimod does not interact with hormonal contraception and no human studies have found any evidence in reducing fertility or increasing miscarriage rates or congenital malformations.[44] Fingolimod is not recommended during pregnancy due to its cardiovascular or musculoskeletal malformations. Fingolimod acts on the receptors responsible for vascular system formation during the period of embryogenesis.[40] It is also contraindicated during breastfeeding. Fingolimod must be stopped 2 months before planning for pregnancy and should be stopped immediately in case of an unplanned pregnancy.[49] When women with MS become pregnant on fingolimod, it must be treated as high risk, and an anomaly scan is recommended.

Dimethyl Fumarate

Although dimethyl fumarate (DMF) does not reduce the effectiveness of hormonal contraception, it can cause gastrointestinal upset which can interfere with the absorption of oral contraceptives.[44] Hence, additional contraceptive measures should be advised during the initial period. A study in rats with the highest tested dose showed evidence of delayed ossification and sexual maturity, low birth, and testicular weight.[50] However, none of the human studies have shown any evidence of reduced fertility or increased congenital malformations or miscarriage rates.[51] As there is limited data regarding the safety of DMF in pregnancy, it is recommended that women with MS use contraception. In case of pregnancy, DMF must be continued only if the benefit outweighs the risk. If planning for pregnancy, MS patients on DMF must be given the option of switching over to another DMT. DMF does not require a washout period because of its short half-life (approximately 1 hour). Due to a lack of enough data, breastfeeding is not recommended.[52]

Teriflunomide

Teriflunomide, a dihydroorotate dehydrogenase inhibitor, is contraindicated during pregnancy as various animal studies demonstrated teratogenicity at equivalent doses to those given to humans.[44] Although the half-life of teriflunomide is 16–18 days, it may remain in the system for up to 2 years due to its long enterohepatic circulation. Hence, women who are planning for conception should stop the medicine and undergo an accelerated elimination procedure. The elimination procedure can be done through the administration of cholestyramine or activated charcoal for a few days until the drug concentration falls to 0.02 mg/dL. It is recommended to continue contraceptive measures for a minimum of 6 weeks after the serum drug concentrations are <0.02 mg/dL on at least two occasions that have been measured 2 weeks apart.[44] Drug elimination procedures should be done in men also as the drug is detected in semen. Women with MS on teriflunomide should not breastfeed as the drug is secreted into the breast milk.[52]

Anti-CD-20 Therapies

Anti-CD-20 mAb therapies for MS include fully humanized glycosylated IgG1 mAb ocrelizumab and ofatumumab, glycoengineered IgG1 chimeric mAb ublituximab, and IgG1 mouse-human chimeric mAb rituximab (RTX).[53] There is very limited data regarding the use of ocrelizumab in pregnancy. Ocrelizumab does not interact with hormonal contraception. The manufacturers recommend the use of contraception in women while receiving ocrelizumab and up to 12 months after the last infusion. The ocrelizumab pregnancy registry consisting of 1,223 recorded pregnancies in women with relapsing remitting multiple sclerosis (RRMS) consisted of 414 women exposed to ocrelizumab within 3 months of conception and 128 women during their first trimester. Seven major congenital anomalies were reported among the 604 pregnancies of known outcome. Among those exposed within 3 months of conception or during the first trimester, there were 171 live births (72.5%), 30 terminations of pregnancy (12.7%), 29 spontaneous miscarriages (12.3%), 4 stillbirths (1.7%), and 2 ectopic pregnancies (2.8%).[54] As immunoglobulins cross the placenta, fetal exposure is likely if the drug is given during pregnancy. Transient

B-cell depletion and lymphopenia up to 6 months after delivery have been reported in both animal and human fetuses after exposure to RTX during pregnancy.[55] It can be presumed that the same may be true with ocrelizumab. Given this, infants should be monitored for B-cell depletion. Live and live-attenuated vaccines should be postponed until there is a recovery in the B-cell count of the infant. A retrospective cohort study of 74 pregnancies among 55 women treated with RTX for MS did not observe any increase in adverse pregnancy outcomes compared with expected national incidence rates and significantly less disease activity, particularly when compared with periconceptional natalizumab-treated cohorts.[56] In the same study, among the 38 live births, most babies were breastfed (89% of the babies) and 8 babies (22%) were still being breastfed when their mothers resumed RTX infusions.[56] The Association of British Neurologists MS Advisory team recommends that anti-CD-20 therapies can be safely given while breastfeeding.[57] Pregnancy data to guide ofatumumab use in pregnancy is very limited and further studies are warranted.[57]

Alemtuzumab

Alemtuzumab, an anti-CD-52 antibody, is a humanized IgG1 mAb that does not impair the effectiveness of hormonal contraception. The serum concentrations of alemtuzumab will be almost undetectable in the plasma a month after the last dose of alemtuzumab.[44] Women with MS on alemtuzumab are advised not to conceive for at least 4 months after the discontinuation of the drug.[45] As there is a risk of autoimmune thyroid disease up to 4 years after the last cycle of alemtuzumab, there is a risk of antibodies against thyroid-stimulating hormone receptors crossing the placenta and inducing transient neonatal Graves' disease.[44] Hence, it is vital to monitor thyroid function tests regularly. The obstetric team must be aware of these risks to ensure adequate precautions and care. Women with MS should not breastfeed during the treatment or within 4 months of receiving the last dose of alemtuzumab.[58]

The details regarding the use of other DMTs during pregnancy have been compiled in **Table 1**.

Delivery and Anesthetic Options in Multiple Sclerosis

Despite few studies demonstrating that maternal pelvis floor function is not affected in patients with MS, the frequency of cesarean section is more, probably due to the fewer gestational weeks and lower fetal birth weight.[59,60] MS must not interfere with the choice of delivery method, either vaginal delivery or cesarean section. The decision should be taken primarily based on the obstetric factors.[61] For patients with MS having sensory deficits that prevent them from recognizing the onset of labor, they must be trained to recognize other symptoms such as increased spasticity, gastrointestinal distress, flushing, and backache which also indicate the onset of labor.[40] During the time of labor, spasticity can be managed by administering benzodiazepines and/or epidural anesthesia. Two large retrospective studies have observed that with regard to the use of anesthesia during labor, spinal, epidural, or spinal-epidural do not increase the disease activity and are considered to be safe in patients with MS.[62,63] A 10-year retrospective study involving 70 pregnancies with MS did not show any significant differences between cesarean and vaginal delivery, and the choice of pain management did not have any influence on the MS activity 6 months after delivery.

Postpartum Care in Multiple Sclerosis

All patients with MS should be encouraged to exclusively breastfeed, although there

TABLE 1: Application of disease-modifying therapies in pregnancy and breastfeeding and need for contraception.[34]

Drug	Guidelines for use during pregnancy		Guidelines for use during breastfeeding		Need for contraception	
	US FDA	EMA	US FDA	EMA	US FDA	EMA
Interferon beta	Data do not indicate a drug-associated risk of birth defects	Can be used in pregnancy if clinically needed	Consider clinical needs and potential adverse effects	Can be used during breastfeeding	No need for contraception indicated	No need for contraception indicated
Glatiramer acetate	Not enough data to provide recommendation	Continue if potential benefit justifies potential risk to fetus	Consider clinical needs and potential adverse effects	Can be used during breastfeeding	No need for contraception indicated	No need for contraception indicated
Dimethyl fumarate	Not enough data to provide recommendation	Continue if potential benefit justifies potential risk to fetus	Consider clinical needs and potential adverse effects	Discontinue while breastfeeding	No need for contraception indicated	Use of contraception is recommended
Teriflunomide	Contraindicated	Contraindicated	Contraindicated	Contraindicated	Use contraception during the treatment and after the last dose, until blood plasma concentration is <0.02 mg/L	Use contraception during the treatment and after the last dose, until blood plasma concentration is <0.02 mg/L
Oral cladribine	Contraindicated	Contraindicated	Contraindicated during breast-feeding and for at least 1 week after the last dose	Contraindicated during breastfeeding and for at least 1 week after the last dose	Use contraception during and for 6 months after treatment	Use contraception during and for 6 months after treatment
Fingolimod	Patients encouraged to avoid pregnancy	Contraindicated	Consider clinical needs and potential adverse effects	Contraindicated	Use contraception during and for 2 months after treatment	Use contraception during and for 2 months after treatment

Continued

Continued

Drug	Guidelines for use during pregnancy		Guidelines for use during breastfeeding		Need for contraception	
	US FDA	EMA	US FDA	EMA	US FDA	EMA
Ozanimod	Patients encouraged to avoid pregnancy	Contraindicated	Consider clinical needs and potential adverse effects	Contraindicated	Use contraception during and for 3 months after treatment	Use contraception during and for 3 months after treatment
Siponimod	Contraindicated	Contraindicated	Consider clinical needs and potential adverse effects	Contraindicated	Use contraception during and for 10 days after treatment	Use contraception during and for 10 days after treatment
Ponesimod	Patients encouraged to avoid pregnancy	Contraindicated	Consider clinical needs and potential adverse effects	Contraindicated	Use contraception during and for 1 week after treatment	Use contraception during and for 1 week after treatment
Alemtuzumab	Not enough data to provide recommendation	Continue if potential benefit justifies potential risk to fetus	Consider clinical needs and potential adverse effects	Contraindicated during breastfeeding and for 4 months after the last dose	Use contraception during and for 4 months after treatment	Use contraception during and for 4 months after treatment
Natalizumab	Not enough data to provide recommendation	Continue if potential benefit justifies potential risk to fetus	Consider clinical needs and potential adverse effects	Should be discontinued during breastfeeding	No need for contraception indicated	No need for contraception indicated
Rituximab	Continue if potential benefit justifies potential risk to fetus	Continue if potential benefit justifies potential risk to fetus	Discontinue during breastfeeding and for 6 months after last dose	Discontinue during breastfeeding and for 6 months after last dose	Use contraception during and for 12 months after treatment	Use contraception during and for 12 months after treatment

Continued

Continued

Drug	Guidelines for use during pregnancy		Guidelines for use during breastfeeding		Need for contraception	
	US FDA	EMA	US FDA	EMA	US FDA	EMA
Ocrelizumab	Not enough data to provide recommendation	Continue if potential benefit justifies potential risk to fetus	Consider clinical needs and potential adverse effects	Discontinue during breastfeeding	Use contraception during and for 6 months after treatment	Use contraception during and for 12 months after treatment
Ofatumumab	Not enough data to provide recommendation	Continue if potential benefit justifies potential risk to fetus	Consider clinical needs and potential adverse effects	Can be used after few days postpartum if clinically needed. If receiving ofatumumab up to the last few months of pregnancy, breastfeeding can be started immediately	Use contraception during and for 6 months after treatment	Use contraception during and for 6 months after treatment
Ublituximab	No safety data on the use of ublituximab in pregnant women	Avoid unless potential benefit justifies potential risk to fetus	Consider clinical needs and potential adverse effects	Can be used after few days postpartum if clinically needed	Use contraception during and for 6 months after treatment	Use contraception during and for 6 months after treatment

(EMA: European Medicines Agency; US FDA: United States Food and Drug Administration) are uncertainties about whether exclusive breastfeeding can reduce the postpartum relapse rate.[64] Storing supplies of breastmilk in the freezer can be considered in case of relapse-associated disability or fatigue or if there is a need to prescribe a medicine not compatible with breastfeeding.[44] There are contraindications for breastfeeding if the patient requires methylprednisolone for postpartum relapses. However, a minimum of 4-hour interruption is recommended between the drug infusion and breastfeeding.[49] Postpartum women with MS should continue taking vitamin D supplementations and their infants should be given vitamin D as per the protocol. Mothers and fathers with MS are at risk of developing depression in the postpartum period. The patients should be made aware of this and advice should be sought when necessary. There is no sufficient evidence to recommend routine umbilical cord blood collection and banking for women with MS for future MS-related treatments (e.g., stem cell therapies).[44]

There is an increase in the risk of relapse after delivery and MS activity is believed to go back to the prepregnancy levels, which can be explained by the sudden change in the hormonal levels after delivery. Hence, it is important to start DMT in the postpartum period, especially for those with a high risk of rebound such as natalizumab, fingolimod, and DMF. DMTs have to be adjusted as per breastfeeding.

AQUAPORIN-4 POSITIVE NEUROMYELITIS OPTICA SPECTRUM DISORDER

Pregnancy and Neuromyelitis Optica Spectrum Disorder: What We Know?

Aquaporin-4 positive NMOSD is predominantly a humoral immunity-mediated disease. Pregnancy induces various immunological and hormonal changes, including a major shift from Th1-mediated to Th2-mediated immunity.[65,66] A shift toward Th2 in pregnancy can lead to increased antigen stimulation and production of AQP4-IgG.[67] Another reason could be the higher levels of estrogen which increase gradually during pregnancy, reaching their peak in the third trimester. Estrogen increases the expression of activation-induced cytidine deaminase (AID), which is responsible for immunoglobulin production.[6,68] and thereby can lead to higher AQP4+ antibody production **(Flowchart 3)**. This is in contrast to what happens in MS, where the shift from Th1-mediated to Th-2 mediated immunity is protective during pregnancy.

The relapse rate increases in the postpartum period (two- to threefold), especially in the first postpartum trimester and for the reasons listed earlier, it has been suggested that it also possibly increases during pregnancy.[7,8,69-71] However, the available data is insufficient to define the relapse risk during pregnancy at present. Higher levels of AQP4+ antibody titers, recent disease activity, especially in the prepregnancy year, and discontinued immunosuppressive treatment have been proposed as risk factors for NMOSD attacks during or soon after pregnancy.[8,72,73]

Women with AQP4+ NMOSD also appear to be at a higher risk of miscarriage compared to the general population.[9] AQP4 is widely expressed in the placental syncytiotrophoblast and levels are highest in the second trimester.[72,74] It has been theorized that the maternal AQP4 antibody can bind to the AQP4 receptors in the placenta and induce placentitis leading to fetal death. However, it is not yet entirely clear to what extent AQP4-IgG contributes to its pathophysiology. Pregnant women with AQP4+ NMOSD have also been found to have a higher incidence of preeclampsia, additionally contributing to adverse pregnancy outcomes.[7,9,75]

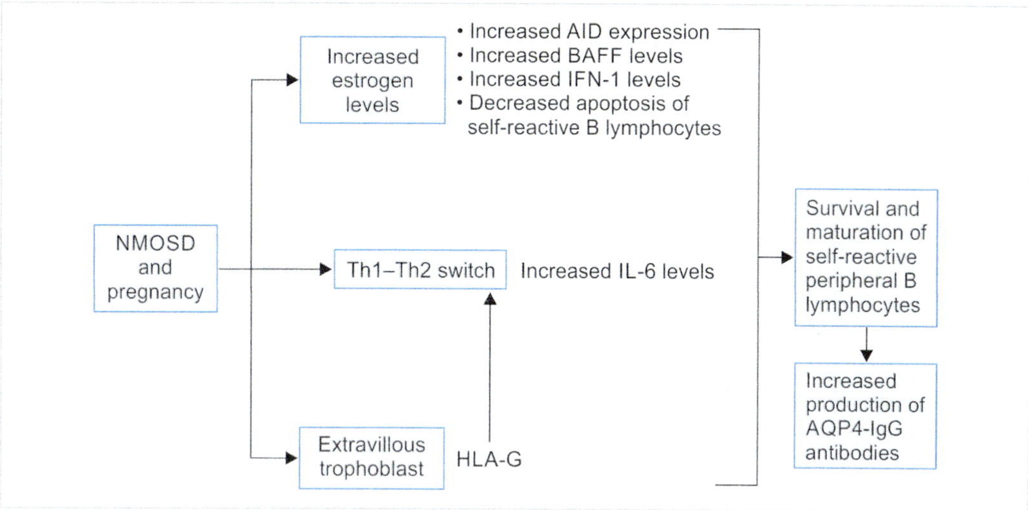

FLOWCHART 3: Immunological and hormonal changes seen during pregnancy in patients with AQP4+ NMOSD.

(AID: activation-induced cytidine deaminase; AQP4: aquaporin-4; BAFF: B-cell activating factor; HLA-G: human leukocyte antigen G; IFN-1: interferon 1; IgG: immunoglobulin G; IL: interleukin; NMOSD: neuromyelitis optica spectrum disorder; Th: T helper cells)

As mentioned earlier, pregnancy outcomes can also be affected by coexisting autoimmune and connective tissue disorders or adverse effects of immunosuppressive treatments administered to patients. Pregnancy in NMOSD women is considered a high-risk pregnancy and therefore, it is extremely important to monitor the patient throughout pregnancy and offer assistance at every step.

Antepartum Planning

Pregnancy is not contraindicated in patients with NMOSD and this should be emphasized to the patient from the initial diagnosis and subsequently thereafter, at each follow-up. Understandably, NMOSD patients are anxious and often tend to avoid or postpone pregnancy. In this respect, it is advised to regularly discuss pregnancy and contraception with the patient, allay the patient's anxiety, and provide answers to all questions as best as possible. As per the 2022 recommendations, pregnancy planning should be favored during a period of inactivity of the disease for at least 12 months and the patient's plans for pregnancy should be borne in mind prior to initiation of DMT.[76] As NMOSD has more severe and disabling relapses, it is recommended to maintain the DMT at least until conception.[76]

Each visit should highlight the patient's desires, discuss disease management, stress on treatment compliance, provide adjustments or modifications of treatment if required, and update their vaccination status. The same recommendations for antenatal vitamin supplementation apply to women with NMOSD as in the general population.

The evidence is not sufficient to make recommendations regarding ART in women with NMOSD. However, in case it is being planned, the risks and benefits of the procedure needs to be evaluated at an individual basis.

During Pregnancy

As pregnancy in women with NMOSD is considered high risk, a multidisciplinary approach toward their management, predominantly involving the neurologist, gynecologist-obstetrician, and the rehabilitation team, should be adopted early on.

The following recommendations are adapted from the French cohort:[76]

- *Follow-up visits during pregnancy*: It is advised that follow-up visits should be solely carried out by obstetricians every month along with a monthly ultrasound.
- *MRI during pregnancy*: Regular follow-up MRIs are not indicated in NMOSD as the disease does not typically show progression between relapses as in MS. There are no studies regarding MRI and pregnancy in women with NMOSD; however, when indicated, especially during an active relapse, MRI can be carried out during pregnancy as per recommendations of the general population. If gadolinium is absolutely essential, it can be administered in any trimester, taking care to avoid linear gadolinium salts.[76]
- *Vaccines*: As there is no specific literature for vaccines in women with NMOSD, general recommendations are borrowed from the management of MS patients. The vaccination status of women with NMOSD should be regularly updated whenever possible; however, treatment should not be delayed pending the administration of vaccines.

Live-attenuated vaccines are contraindicated during pregnancy and should be avoided in the month before conception. Measles, mumps, and rubella (MMR), chicken pox, and pertussis vaccines should be completed before pregnancy or in the postpartum period before starting immunosuppressive treatments. Inactivated vaccines such as influenza and coronavirus disease 2019 (COVID-19) can be administered regardless of the trimester of pregnancy, when indicated.

All vaccines can be administered in the postpartum period except yellow fever vaccine which is contraindicated during breastfeeding.

Disease-modifying Therapy Use during Pregnancy

Azathioprine (AZA): AZA, a purine synthesis inhibitor, causes decreased proliferation of lymphocytes and thereby immunosuppression. Most of the evidence comes from AZA use in women with other inflammatory and autoimmune disorders. It is considered a relatively safe option during pregnancy as most human studies and meta-analyses have failed to show any significant association between AZA exposure and risk of major congenital malformations.[72,76-79] There were some concerns about low birth weight, premature birth, and cardiac septal defects following administration of AZA; however, it is likely that these findings were confounded by the underlying diseases of the mother.[80] Therefore, its use can be considered during pregnancy after careful risk-benefit evaluation.

Mycophenolate mofetil (MMF) and methotrexate are teratogenic and contraindicated in pregnancy. Reliable contraception should be used during the use of these treatments and their initiation should preferably be avoided in women of childbearing age. In case of use, MMF should be stopped at least 6 weeks and methotrexate at least 6 months before conception and alternative treatments should be considered.[72]

RTX: An anti-CD-20 mAb and B-cell depletor, RTX has long been used as an effective option in the treatment of patients with NMOSD. In a systematic review of 102 pregnancies in women with MS and NMOSD and RTX use within 6 months of conception, no major safety signal was identified.[81] No effects on fertility have been reported.

Monoclonal antibodies, being large molecules, do not cross the placenta in the first trimester of pregnancy but begin to do so in the second and third trimesters. Transient B-cell depletion can be seen in newborns which is usually reversible within 6 months of birth.[81] Vaccination schedules should then be modified accordingly.

Initial recommendation was a 12-month washout period after the last dose of RTX. However, many experts consider conception soon after the last infusion acceptable after thorough risk-benefit evaluation.[72] We recommend the last infusion at least a month before conception to reduce the chance of fetal exposure and provide optimal protection to the mother during pregnancy. Redosing should be considered if a severe relapse occurs during pregnancy.

Tocilizumab (TCZ): A humanized mAb, against interleukin 6 (IL-6) receptor, has been used in severe cases of NMOSD. There is no data on pregnant women with NMOSD and the use of TCZ. Animal studies have shown no teratogenicity. Studying its use in patients with rheumatoid arthritis, there was slight increased risk of miscarriage and premature births reported, but the results may have been biased by the concomitant use of methotrexate in nearly 20% of patients.[82] No significant increase in the risk of congenital anomalies was reported.

The current guidelines recommend TCZ should be stopped 3 months before conception, but experts have suggested that TCZ can be continued until and during pregnancy in patients with very severe NMOSD.[72]

Newer Food and Drug Administration-approved Therapies

Eculizumab (ECZ): Most of the data comes from the use of ECZ, a C5 inhibitor, in paroxysmal nocturnal hemoglobinuria (PNH) and other hematological syndromes. The use of ECZ in pregnant women has been described in these disorders and no major adverse outcomes were flagged off.[83] Though there is no data on women with NMOSD, it can serve as a potential option during pregnancy in severe NMOSD based on an individual assessment of risk and safety profile.

Satralizumab and inebilizumab: Currently, literature is lacking regarding the use of satralizumab and inebilizumab in pregnant women with NMOSD. Owing to its similarity to TCZ, satralizumab is not expected to have potent teratogenic effects in humans. Recently, a case was published from Japan where an AQP4+ NMOSD patient safely completed pregnancy, delivery, and breastfeeding under satralizumab treatment.[84]

Similarly, inebilizumab, a CD-19 mAb and B-cell-depleting agent, is expected to have similar effects as RTX. The effect of these antibodies on pregnancy outcomes remains to be investigated.

Intrapartum delivery and anesthesia: Owing to limited data, the same recommendations for the mode of delivery and obstetrical anesthesia apply as in the general population, where obstetrical indications guide the abovementioned decisions. The increased risk of preeclampsia should be noted in these patients.

Postpartum Period and Breastfeeding

Breastfeeding is not contraindicated in patients with NMOSD. However, the neurologist, obstetrician, pediatrician, and the patient need to discuss strategies depending on the patient's disease activity and desires.

There is no role for specific preventative treatments to prevent postpartum relapses in NMOSD. Due to the high risk of postpartum relapses, their severity, and ensuing disability, it is best to resume immunomodulatory treatments soon after delivery, if they were interrupted during pregnancy, according to patient's wishes, breastfeeding status, indications, and contraindications of individual treatments.

In case of breastfeeding, AZA and mAbs such as RTX and ECZ are potentially safer choices in these patients along with careful monitoring.[72] As stated earlier, transient B-cell depletion can be seen in newborns of mothers on B-cell depleting therapies and therefore, vaccination should be planned accordingly.

Immunoglobulin G antibodies cross the placenta in the second and third trimester of pregnancy and AQP4-IgG is likely to be transferred to the fetus. Measured serum levels of AQP4-IgG in the umbilical cord blood at birth were high in newborns of mothers with active NMOSD during pregnancy; however, they turned seronegative by 1-3 months of age and they showed no clinical symptoms of NMOSD.[8,85]

Treatment of Relapses during Pregnancy and Breastfeeding

As in MS, IVMP for a short course (1,000 mg/day for 3-5 days) can be administered during an active relapse. The evidence for the association between cleft palate and corticosteroids in humans is questionable.[86,87] However, due to a possible low risk during the first trimester, its use must be limited following a risk-benefit analysis.[72] Fluorinated corticosteroids such as dexamethasone, betamethasone, and triamcinolone pose a higher risk and should be avoided.

The transfer of high doses of IVMP in breast milk has been found to be only about 1% of the maternal amount. Breastfeeding mothers can be administered methylprednisolone, preferably about 4 hours after the oral dose or at the end of infusion. No adverse outcomes were observed after 3-12 months of follow-up in infants who were breastfed 4 hours after the infusion.[88]

Plasmapheresis (PLEX) or immunoadsorption can be carried out with the same risks during and outside of pregnancy. It is however important to note that in rhesus immunoglobulin-D (RhD)-negative mothers, PLEX would remove the administered anti-D immunoglobulins.[72] Though intravenous immunoglobulin (IVIG) is well tolerated, owing to the lack of definite evidence for its use in treating acute relapses in AQP4+ NMOSD, it is not routinely recommended, and perhaps maybe preserved for treatment-refractory cases or where steroids/PLEX are contraindicated.[76]

MYELIN OLIGODENDROCYTE GLYCOPROTEIN ANTIBODY-ASSOCIATED DISEASE

Myelin oligodendrocyte glycoprotein antibody-associated disease is a distinct oligodendrocytopathy and CNS demyelinating disorder. It can have a monophasic or relapsing course with varied presentations affecting different parts of the neuraxis.[89] Though the attacks can be as severe as in NMOSD, patients tend to have a better recovery.

Myelin oligodendrocyte glycoprotein antibody-associated disease patients do not show any gender predilection and the disease typically presents in young adults, although a significant proportion of patients develop the condition in childhood.[90]

Considering that the disease starts young in many patients, it is important that treating pediatricians are aware of the impact the disease, choice of treatment, and the decisions can have in the future. It is always important to involve the patient and their caregivers in a shared decision-making approach. No studies or case reports have discussed the effect of MOGAD on fertility yet.

The literature regarding MOGAD and pregnancy is sparse at present with few retrospective studies providing some specific data.[73,91] Studies found an increase in ARR during the postpartum period compared to pregnancy. One of them noted a decrease in ARR during pregnancy compared to the prepregnancy period; however, another study did not find any significant change.[73,91] The evidence is currently not sufficient to make any formal conclusions.

Data on pregnancy outcomes in patients with MOGAD are limited, although risks seem to be decreased as compared to patients with AQP4+ NMOSD.[92] In a recent retrospective analysis of 25 pregnancies in patients with MOGAD, only a single miscarriage and two preterm births were identified, which were similar to those observed in the general population.[93] There is not enough data regarding congenital malformations or neonatal complications.

Most of the guidelines for management of pregnancy in MOGAD are derived from the previously described NMOSD studies and follow similar recommendations. Prednisolone is not contraindicated and can be maintained during pregnancy. AZA, RTX, and TCZ remain viable options until and during pregnancy, and their use should be individualized based on severity of disease, risks, and benefits. During a relapse, high-dose intravenous corticosteroids, IVIG, and apheresis can all be considered. IVIG is generally considered safe during pregnancy; however, there is a possible risk of maternal hypovolemia, hyperviscosity, and subsequent thromboembolism, especially when used as maintenance IVIG and therefore, the patient needs to be kept under surveillance.[92]

DUAL-SERONEGATIVE NEUROMYELITIS OPTICA SPECTRUM DISORDER

Dual-seronegative NMOSD, negative for both AQP4-igG and MOG-IgG antibodies, is probably the least represented group in studies dealing with NMOSD and pregnancy. Studies often combine seropositive and seronegative patients and therefore, not much is known solely about this group. In one study, the ARR was lower during pregnancy compared to the prepregnancy period.[91] However, the data is severely lacking to make any conclusions.

For now, similar recommendations apply to this group as the seropositive NMOSD group till we have more information.

CONCLUSION

Pregnancy induces various immunological and hormonal changes, including a major shift from Th1-mediated to Th2-mediated immunity. This is protective during pregnancy in MS. However, higher estrogen levels and a shift toward Th2 in pregnancy can lead to increased antigen stimulation and production of AQP4-IgG in NMOSD.

The relationship between MS and pregnancy is a complex and important topic. MS is generally considered not to affect a woman's ability to conceive and carry a pregnancy to term. It does not increase the rates of premature birth, stillbirth, birth defects, cesarean deliveries, or spontaneous abortions. Pregnancy often significantly reduces disease activity, although some patients may experience severe relapses during pregnancy. Emerging data suggest that delaying the initiation of DMTs or stopping these medications before or immediately after conception is linked to a higher relapse rate during pregnancy. It is important to consider future pregnancies when prescribing disease-modifying drugs to women of childbearing age. If a relapse occurs, corticosteroids can be administered during pregnancy and breastfeeding. MS does not inherently make pregnancy high risk and should not limit delivery options.

The available research in NMOSD, MOGAD, and pregnancy remains much lower compared to MS. Higher levels of AQP4+ antibody titers, recent disease activity, especially in the prepregnancy year, and discontinued immunosuppressive treatment have been proposed as risk factors for NMOSD attacks during or soon after pregnancy. Women with AQP4+ NMOSD also appear to be at a higher risk of miscarriage and preeclampsia compared to the general population. Continuation of appropriate DMT during pregnancy should be considered based on prepregnancy severity. Breastfeeding is not contraindicated in patients with NMOSD. Due to the high risk of postpartum relapses, it is prudent to resume immunomodulatory treatments soon after delivery unless contraindicated. Most of the guidelines for management of pregnancy in MOGAD are derived from NMOSD literature and largely follow similar recommendations at present.

The recent efforts to compile and provide evidence-based recommendations are a step in the right direction. Much work is required to further our understanding in the field and fill the existing knowledge gaps. As pregnant women are often excluded from clinical trials, there is a critical need for more comprehensive pregnancy registries and studies to evaluate the risks of DMTs during pregnancy and lactation. These registries should be created to monitor pregnancies and DMT use, its effects, and outcomes on both mother and child. Physicians and neurologists should be encouraged to include patients in these registries. Pregnant women and their caregivers should also have the option to self-enroll to increase participation. We hope to continue our efforts in this direction, to reevaluate the recommendations periodically, and to provide guidance applicable to the Indian context.

REFERENCES

1. Levin S, Rimmer K, Vargas WS. Neuroimmunologic disorders in pregnancy. Handb Clin Neurol. 2020;172:105-23.
2. Douglass LH, Jorgensen CL. Pregnancy and multiple sclerosis. Am J Obstet Gynecol. 1948;55:332-6.
3. Confavreux C, Hutchinson M, Hours MM, Cortinovis-Tourniaire P, Moreau T. Rate of pregnancy-related relapse in multiple sclerosis. Pregnancy in Multiple Sclerosis Group. N Engl J Med. 1998;339:285-91.
4. Vukusic S, Hutchinson M, Hours M, Moreau T, Cortinovis-Tourniaire P, Adeleine P, et al. Pregnancy and multiple sclerosis (the PRIMS study): clinical predictors of post-partum relapse. Brain J Neurol. 2004;127:1353-60.
5. Voskuhl R, Momtazee C. Pregnancy: Effect on Multiple Sclerosis, Treatment Considerations, and Breastfeeding. Neurother J Am Soc Exp Neurother. 2017;14:974-84.
6. Davoudi V, Keyhanian K, Bove RM, Chitnis T. Immunology of neuromyelitis optica during pregnancy. Neurol Neuroimmunol Neuroinflamm. 2016;3:e288.
7. Klawiter EC, Bove R, Elsone L, Alvarez E, Borisow N, Cortez M, et al. High risk of postpartum relapses in neuromyelitis optica spectrum disorder. Neurology. 2017;89:2238-44.
8. Shimizu Y, Fujihara K, Ohashi T, Nakashima I, Yokoyama K, Ikeguch R, et al. Pregnancy-related relapse risk factors in women with anti-AQP4 antibody positivity and neuromyelitis optica spectrum disorder. Mult Scler. 2016;22:1413-20.
9. Nour MM, Nakashima I, Coutinho E, Woodhall M, Sousa F, Revis J, et al. Pregnancy outcomes in aquaporin-4-positive neuromyelitis optica spectrum disorder. Neurology. 2016;86:79-87.
10. Jarius S, Ruprecht K, Wildemann B, Kuempfel T, Ringelstein M, Geis C, et al. Contrasting disease patterns in seropositive and seronegative neuromyelitis optica: A multicentre study of 175 patients. J Neuroinflamm. 2012;9:14.
11. Ferreira LMR, Meissner TB, Tilburgs T, Strominger JL. HLA-G: At the Interface of Maternal–Fetal Tolerance. Trends Immunol. 2017;38:272-86.
12. Blanco O, Tirado I, Muñoz-Fernández R, Abadía-Molina AC, García-Pacheco JM, Peña J, et al. Human decidual stromal cells express HLA-G:

Effects of cytokines and decidualization. Hum Reprod Oxf Engl. 2008;23:144-52.
13. Kovats S, Main EK, Librach C, Stubblebine M, Fisher SJ, DeMars R. A class I antigen, HLA-G, expressed in human trophoblasts. Science. 1990;248:220-3.
14. van der Meer A, Lukassen HGM, van Lierop MJC, Wijnands F, Mosselman S, Braat DDM, et al. Membrane-bound HLA-G activates proliferation and interferon-gamma production by uterine natural killer cells. Mol Hum Reprod. 2004;10: 189-95.
15. Nahum R, Brenner O, Zahalka MA, Traub L, Quintana F, Moroz C. Blocking of the placental immune-modulatory ferritin activates Th1 type cytokines and affects placenta development, fetal growth and the pregnancy outcome. Hum Reprod Oxf Engl. 2004;19:715-22.
16. Wegmann TG, Lin H, Guilbert L, Mosmann TR. Bidirectional cytokine interactions in the maternal-fetal relationship: is successful pregnancy a TH2 phenomenon? Immunol Today. 1993;14:353-6.
17. Fuhler GM. The immune system and microbiome in pregnancy. Best Pract Res Clin Gastroenterol. 2020;44-45:101671.
18. Kumar P, Magon N. Hormones in pregnancy. Niger Med J Niger Med Assoc. 2012;53:179-83.
19. Hemmer B, Kerschensteiner M, Korn T. Role of the innate and adaptive immune responses in the course of multiple sclerosis. Lancet Neurol. 2015;14:406-19.
20. Soldan SS, Alvarez Retuerto AI, Sicotte NL, Voskuhl RR. Immune modulation in multiple sclerosis patients treated with the pregnancy hormone estriol. J Immunol. 2003;171:6267-74.
21. Raghupathy R, Kalinka J. Cytokine imbalance in pregnancy complications and its modulation. Front Biosci J Virtual Libr. 2008;13:985-94.
22. Vukusic S, Confavreux C. Pregnancy and multiple sclerosis: the children of PRIMS. Clin Neurol Neurosurg. 2006;108:266-70.
23. Rossi C, Cicalini I, Zucchelli M, di Ioia M, Onofrj M, Federici L, et al. Metabolomic Signature in Sera of Multiple Sclerosis Patients during Pregnancy. Int J Mol Sci. 2018;19:3589.
24. Houtchens MK, Edwards NC, Phillips AL. Relapses and disease-modifying drug treatment in pregnancy and live birth in US women with MS. Neurology. 2018;91:e1570-8.
25. Mendibe Bilbao M, Boyero Durán S, Bárcena Llona J, Rodriguez-Antigüedad A. Multiple sclerosis: Pregnancy and women's health issues. Neurologia. 2019;34:259-69.
26. Coyle PK, Oh J, Magyari M, Oreja-Guevara C, Houtchens M. Management strategies for female patients of reproductive potential with multiple sclerosis: An evidence-based review. Mult Scler Relat Disord. 2019;32:54-63.
27. Rankin K, Bove R. Caring for Women with Multiple Sclerosis Across the Lifespan. Curr Neurol Neurosci Rep. 2018;18:36.
28. González-Madrid E, Rangel-Ramírez MA, Mendoza-León MJ, Álvarez-Mardones O, González PA, Kalergis AM, et al. Risk Factors from Pregnancy to Adulthood in Multiple Sclerosis Outcome. Int J Mol Sci. 2022;23:7080.
29. Mohammadi M, Abdi M, Alidadi M, Mohamed W, Zibara K, Ragerdi Kashani I. Medroxyprogesterone acetate attenuates demyelination, modulating microglia activation, in a cuprizone neurotoxic demyelinating mouse model. Am J Neurodegener Dis. 2021;10:57-68.
30. Curtis KM, Tepper NK, Jatlaoui TC, Berry-Bibee E, Horton LG, Zapata LB, et al. U.S. Medical Eligibility Criteria for Contraceptive Use, 2016. MMWR Recomm Rep. 2016;65:1-103.
31. Kim D, Leurer C, So B, Casserly C, Seyman E, Baral S, et al. Sexual Dysfunction in Multiple Sclerosis: A Systematic Review and Meta-analysis of Prevalence (P5.2-089). Neurology. 2019;92:P5. 2-089.
32. Coyle PK. Management of women with multiple sclerosis through pregnancy and after childbirth. Ther Adv Neurol Disord. 2016;9:198-210.
33. Graham EL, Bakkensen JB, Anderson A, Lancki N, Davidson A, Perez Giraldo G, et al. Inflammatory Activity After Diverse Fertility Treatments: A Multicenter analysis in the Modern Multiple Sclerosis Treatment Era. Neurol Neuroimmunol Neuroinflamm. 2023;10:e200106.
34. Graham EL, Bove R, Costello K, Crayton H, Jacobs DA, Shah S, et al. Practical Considerations for Managing Pregnancy in Patients with Multiple Sclerosis. Neurol Clin Pract. 2024;14(2):e200253.
35. Nesbitt C, Rath L, Zhong M, Cheng AC, Butzkueven H, Wesselingh R, et al. Vaccinations in patients with multiple sclerosis: review and recommendations. Med J Aust. 2021;214:350-4.e1.
36. Reyes S, Ramsay M, Ladhani S, Amirthalingam G, Singh N, Cores C, et al. Protecting people with multiple sclerosis through vaccination. Pract Neurol. 2020;20:435-45.
37. Otero-Romero S, Rodríguez-García J, Vilella A, Ara JR, Brieva L, Calles C, et al. Recommendations for vaccination in patients with multiple sclerosis who are eligible for immunosuppressive therapies:

Spanish consensus statement. Neurologia. 2021; 36:50-60.

38. Ray JG, Vermeulen MJ, Bharatha A, Montanera WJ, Park AL. Association between MRI Exposure during Pregnancy and Fetal and Childhood Outcomes. JAMA. 2016;316(9):952-61.
39. Barrera CA, Francavilla ML, Serai SD, Edgar JC, Jaimes C, Gee MS, et al. Specific Absorption Rate and Specific Energy Dose: Comparison of 1.5-T versus 3.0-T Fetal MRI. Radiology. 2020;295: 664-74.
40. Varytė G, Zakarevičienė J, Ramašauskaitė D, Laužikienė D, Arlauskienė A. Pregnancy and Multiple Sclerosis: An Update on the Disease Modifying Treatment Strategy and a Review of Pregnancy's Impact on Disease Activity. Med Kaunas Lith. 2020;56:49.
41. Medeiros Junior WLG de, Demore CC, Mazaro LP, de Souza MFN, Parolin LF, Melo LH, et al. Urinary tract infection in patients with multiple sclerosis: An overview. Mult Scler Relat Disord. 2020;46:102462.
42. Abdel-Aziz Elzayat M, Barnett-Vanes A, Dabour MFE, Cheng F. Prevalence of undiagnosed asymptomatic bacteriuria and associated risk factors during pregnancy: a cross-sectional study at two tertiary centres in Cairo, Egypt. BMJ Open. 2017;7:e013198.
43. Haensgen H, Albornoz E, Opazo MC, Bugueño K, Jara Fernández EL, Binzberger R, et al. Gestational Hypothyroxinemia Affects its Offspring with a Reduced Suppressive Capacity Impairing the Outcome of the Experimental Autoimmune Encephalomyelitis. Front Immunol. 2018;9:1257.
44. Dobson R, Dassan P, Roberts M, Giovannoni G, Nelson-Piercy C, Brex PA. UK consensus on pregnancy in multiple sclerosis: "Association of British Neurologists" guidelines. Pract Neurol. 2019;19:106-14.
45. Kaplan TB. Management of Demyelinating Disorders in Pregnancy. Neurol Clin. 2019;37:17-30.
46. Portaccio E, Moiola L, Martinelli V, Annovazzi P, Ghezzi A, Zaffaroni M, et al. Pregnancy decision-making in women with multiple sclerosis treated with natalizumab: II: Maternal risks. Neurology. 2018;90:e832-9.
47. Zhovtis Ryerson L, Frohman TC, Foley J, Kister I, Weinstock-Guttman B, Tornatore C, et al. Extended interval dosing of natalizumab in multiple sclerosis. J Neurol Neurosurg Psychiatry. 2016;87: 885-9.
48. Baker TE, Cooper SD, Kessler L, Hale TW. Transfer of natalizumab into breast milk in a mother with multiple sclerosis. J Hum Lact. 2015;31:233-6.
49. Bodiguel E, Bensa C, Brassat D, Laplaud D, Le Page E, Ouallet J-C, et al. Multiple sclerosis and pregnancy. Rev Neurol (Paris). 2014;170: 247-65.
50. TECFIDERA (Dimethyl Fumarate) Delayed-Release Capsules, for Oral Use Full Prescribing Information. [online] Available from https://www.tecfidera.com/pdfs/full-prescribing-information.pdf [Last accessed on 22 September 2019].
51. Gold R, Phillips JT, Havrdova E, Bar-Or A, Kappos L, Kim N, et al. Delayed-release Dimethyl Fumarate and Pregnancy: Preclinical Studies and Pregnancy Outcomes from Clinical Trials and Postmarketing Experience. Neurol Ther. 2015;4:93-104.
52. Bove RM, Houtchens MK. Pregnancy Management in Multiple Sclerosis and Other Demyelinating Diseases. Contin Lifelong Learn Neurol. 2022; 28:12.
53. de Sèze J, Maillart E, Gueguen A, Laplaud DA, Michel L, Thouvenot E, et al. Anti-CD20 therapies in multiple sclerosis: From pathology to the clinic. Front Immunol. 2023;14:1004795.
54. ECTRIMS. (2021). The Digital Experience: 37th Congress of the European Committee for Treatment and Research in Multiple Sclerosis. [online] Available from https://www.ectrims-congress.eu/2021.html [Last accessed September, 2024].
55. Chakravarty EF, Murray ER, Kelman A, Farmer P. Pregnancy outcomes after maternal exposure to rituximab. Blood. 2011;117:1499-506.
56. Smith JB, Hellwig K, Fink K, Lyell DJ, Piehl F, Langer-Gould A. Rituximab, MS, and pregnancy. Neurology Neuroimmunol Neuroinflamm. 2020;7(4):e734.
57. Dobson R, Rog D, Ovadia C, Murray K, Hughes S, Ford HL, et al. Anti-CD20 therapies in pregnancy and breast feeding: a review and ABN guidelines. Pract Neurol. 2023;23:6-14.
58. LEMTRADA (Alemtuzumab) Injection, for Intravenous Use. Full Prescribing Information. [online] Available from https://www. products.sanofi.us/Lemtrada/Lemtrada.pdf [Last accessed on 23 September 2019].
59. Lourenço GA, Nogueira LAC, Rocco R, Fragoso YD, Alves-Leon SV. Multiple Sclerosis does not affect the muscular strength of the pelvic floor during pregnancy a case control study. Mult Scler Relat Disord. 2021;49:102746.
60. De Giglio L, Federici S, Ruggieri S, Borriello G, D'Errico Ma, De Angelis C, et al. Cesarean section in women with MS: A choice or a need? Mult Scler Relat Disord. 2020;38:101867.

61. Kaisey M, Sicotte N, Giesser B. Multiple sclerosis management and reproductive changes: A guide for general neurologists. Neurol Clin Pract. 2018;8:142-7.
62. Harazim H, Štourač P, Janků P, Zelinková H, Frank K, Dufek M, et al. Obstetric anesthesia/analgesia does not affect disease course in multiple sclerosis: 10-year retrospective cohort study. Brain Behav. 2018;8:e01082.
63. Lavie C, Rollot F, Durand-Dubief F, Marignier R, Ionescu I, Casey R, et al. Neuraxial analgesia is not associated with an increased risk of post-partum relapses in MS. Mult Scler. 2019;25:591-600.
64. Hellwig K, Rockhoff M, Herbstritt S, Borisow N, Haghikia A, Elias-Hamp B, et al. Exclusive Breastfeeding and the Effect on Postpartum Multiple Sclerosis Relapses. JAMA Neurol. 2015;72(10):1132-8.
65. Qiu K, He Q, Chen X, Liu H, Deng S, Lu W. Pregnancy-related Immune Changes and Demyelinating Diseases of the Central Nervous System. Front Neurol. 2019;10:1070.
66. Perricone C, de Carolis C, Perricone R. Pregnancy and autoimmunity: a common problem. Best Pract Res Clin Rheumatol. 2012;26:47-60.
67. Orsi NM, Tribe RM. Cytokine networks and the regulation of uterine function in pregnancy and parturition. J Neuroendocrinol. 2008;20:462-9.
68. Hsu H-C, Wu Y, Yang P, Wu Q, Job G, Chen J, et al. Overexpression of Activation-induced Cytidine Deaminase in B Cells is Associated with Production of Highly Pathogenic Autoantibodies. J Immunol. 2007;178:5357-65.
69. Bourre B, Marignier R, Zéphir H, Papeix C, Brassat D, Castelnovo G, et al. Neuromyelitis optica and pregnancy. Neurology. 2012;78:875-9.
70. Huang Y, Wang Y, Zhou Y, Huang Q, Sun X, Chen C, et al. Pregnancy in neuromyelitis optica spectrum disorder: A multicenter study from South China. J Neurol Sci. 2017;372:152-6.
71. Kim W, Kim S-H, Nakashima I, Takai Y, Fujihara K, Leite MI, et al. Influence of pregnancy on neuromyelitis optica spectrum disorder. Neurology. 2012;78:1264-7.
72. Mao-Draayer Y, Thiel S, Mills EA, Chitnis T, Fabian M, Katz Sand I, et al. Neuromyelitis optica spectrum disorders and pregnancy: therapeutic considerations. Nat Rev Neurol. 2020;16:154-70.
73. Wang L, Zhou L, ZhangBao J, Huang W, Chang X, Lu C, et al. Neuromyelitis optica spectrum disorder: pregnancy-related attack and predictive risk factors. J Neurol Neurosurg Psychiatry. 2020;92:53-61.
74. Saadoun S, Waters P, Leite MI, Bennett JL, Vincent A, Papadopoulos MC. Neuromyelitis Optica IgG Causes Placental Inflammation and Fetal Death. J Immunol. 2013;191:2999-3005.
75. Fragoso YD, Adoni T, Bichuetti DB, Brooks JBB, Ferreira MLB, Oliveira EML, et al. Neuromyelitis optica and pregnancy. J Neurol. 2013;260:2614-9.
76. Vukusic S, Marignier R, Ciron J, Bourre B, Cohen M, Deschamps R, et al. Pregnancy and neuromyelitis optica spectrum disorders: 2022 recommendations from the French Multiple Sclerosis Society. Mult Scler. 2023;29:37-51.
77. Akbari M, Shah S, Velayos FS, Mahadevan U, Cheifetz AS. Systematic review and meta-analysis on the effects of thiopurines on birth outcomes from female and male patients with inflammatory bowel disease. Inflamm Bowel Dis. 2013;19:15-22.
78. Francella A, Dyan A, Bodian C, Rubin P, Chapman M, Present DH. The safety of 6-mercaptopurine for childbearing patients with inflammatory bowel disease: A retrospective cohort study. Gastroenterology. 2003;124:9-17.
79. Coelho J, Beaugerie L, Colombel JF, Hébuterne X, Lerebours E, Lémann M, et al. Pregnancy outcome in patients with inflammatory bowel disease treated with thiopurines: cohort from the CESAME Study. Gut. 2011;60:198-203.
80. Cleary BJ, Källén B. Early pregnancy azathioprine use and pregnancy outcomes. Birth Defects Res A Clin Mol Teratol. 2009;85:647-54.
81. Das G, Damotte V, Gelfand JM, Bevan C, Cree BAC, Do L, et al. Rituximab before and during pregnancy: A systematic review, and a case series in MS and NMOSD. Neurol Neuroimmunol Neuroinflamm. 2018;5:e453.
82. Hoeltzenbein M, Beck E, Rajwanshi R, Gøtestam Skorpen C, Berber E, Schaefer C, et al. Tocilizumab use in pregnancy: Analysis of a global safety database including data from clinical trials and post-marketing data. Semin Arthritis Rheum. 2016;46:238-45.
83. Sarno L, Tufano A, Maruotti GM, Martinelli P, Balletta MM, Russo D. Eculizumab in pregnancy: a narrative overview. J Nephrol. 2019;32:17-25.
84. Yoshida T, Watanabe O, Nomura M, Yoshimoto Y, Maki Y, Takashima H. Neuromyelitis optica spectrum disorder safely and successfully treated with satralizumab during pregnancy and breastfeeding: a case report. Front Neurol. 2023;14:1322412.
85. Asgari N, Henriksen TB, Petersen T, Lillevang ST, Weinshenker BG. Pregnancy outcomes in a woman with neuromyelitis optica. Neurology. 2014;83:1576-7.

86. Pradat P, Robert-Gnansia E, Di Tanna GL, Rosano A, Lisi A, Mastroiacovo P, et al. First trimester exposure to corticosteroids and oral clefts. Birth Defects Res A Clin Mol Teratol. 2003;67:968-70.
87. Skuladottir H, Wilcox AJ, Ma C, Lammer EJ, Rasmussen SA, Werler MM, et al. Corticosteroid use and risk of orofacial clefts. Birth Defects Res A Clin Mol Teratol. 2014;100:499-506.
88. Boz C, Terzi M, Zengin Karahan S, Sen S, Sarac Y, Emrah Mavis M. Safety of IV pulse methylprednisolone therapy during breastfeeding in patients with multiple sclerosis. Mult Scler J. 2018;24:1205-11.
89. Banwell B, Bennett JL, Marignier R, Kim HJ, Brilot F, Flanagan EP, et al. Diagnosis of myelin oligodendrocyte glycoprotein antibody-associated disease: International MOGAD Panel proposed criteria. Lancet Neurol. 2023;22:268-82.
90. Jurynczyk M, Messina S, Woodhall MR, Raza N, Everett R, Roca-Fernandez A, et al. Clinical presentation and prognosis in MOG-antibody disease: a UK study. Brain J Neurol. 2017;140:3128-38.
91. Collongues N, Alves Do Rego C, Bourre B, Biotti D, Marignier R, da Silva AM, et al. Pregnancy in Patients with AQP4-Ab, MOG-Ab, or Double-Negative Neuromyelitis Optica Disorder. Neurology. 2021;96:e2006-15.
92. Leite MI, Panahloo Z, Harrison N, Palace J. A systematic literature review to examine the considerations around pregnancy in women of child-bearing age with myelin oligodendrocyte glycoprotein antibody-associated disease (MOGAD) or aquaporin 4 neuromyelitis optica spectrum disorder (AQP4+ NMOSD). Mult Scler Relat Disord. 2023:104760.
93. Carra-Dallière C, Rollot F, Deschamps R, Ciron J, Vukusic S, Audoin B, et al. Pregnancy and post-partum in patients with myelin-oligodendrocyte glycoprotein antibody-associated disease. Mult Scler J. 2023;29:270-6.

CHAPTER 12

Symptomatic Management in Patients with Central Nervous System Demyelinating Disorders

AT Prabhakar

ABSTRACT

Central nervous system (CNS) demyelination disorders, like multiple sclerosis (MS), present with a variety of symptoms that can significantly impact patients' quality of life. Effective symptomatic management is crucial to improving daily functioning and overall well-being. This chapter explores comprehensive strategies for managing symptoms associated with CNS demyelination disorders, focusing on pharmacologic, nonpharmacologic, and lifestyle interventions. Emphasis is placed on personalized care, addressing comorbidities, and integrating evidence-based practices to enhance symptom control and patient outcomes.

Keywords: Symptomatic management, Multiple sclerosis (MS), Neuromyelitis optica (NMO).

INTRODUCTION

Central nervous system (CNS) demyelination disorders, primarily represented by multiple sclerosis (MS) and neuromyelitis optica (NMO), are characterized by the immune-mediated destruction of myelin sheaths surrounding nerve fibers. This pathology leads to a range of neurological symptoms that can vary in severity and impact daily life. Symptomatic management is essential in maximizing patient function and independence, complementing disease-modifying therapies.

COMPREHENSIVE APPROACH TO SYMPTOMATIC MANAGEMENT

Key Considerations

- *Distinguishing symptoms:* Differentiating between exacerbations, pseudoexacerbations, and progression of chronic symptoms is critical. Exacerbations are due to new CNS inflammation, pseudoexacerbations are typically triggered by noninflammatory factors, and chronic progression reflects long-term disease evolution.
- *Symptom clusters and comorbidities:* Understanding symptom clusters and their underlying etiologies helps tailor multifactorial treatment plans. Comorbid conditions such as depression, sleep disorders, and vascular diseases can exacerbate MS symptoms and should be addressed concurrently.

Pharmacologic Interventions

Evidence-based Treatments

- *Dalfampridine:* The only Food and Drug Administration (FDA)-approved medication specifically for MS symptom management, primarily used to improve walking speed.[1]

- *Baclofen:* Commonly used for managing spasticity, though their side effects must be carefully monitored. Baclofen pump has been found to be useful is severe spasticity.[2]
- *Antidepressants:* Selective serotonin reuptake inhibitors (SSRIs) and serotonin-norepinephrine reuptake inhibitors (SNRIs) are frequently prescribed for managing depression and anxiety associated with MS.[3]

Emerging Treatments

- *Cannabinoids:* Increasingly studied for their potential benefits in managing spasticity and pain, although regulatory and safety considerations remain.[4]
- *Modafinil and amantadine*: Used for treating fatigue, with varying degrees of efficacy and patient tolerance.[5]

Nonpharmacologic Interventions

Physical Therapy

- *Exercise:* Tailored exercise programs improve mobility, strength, and overall physical health. Aerobic exercises, resistance training, and flexibility routines are recommended based on the patient's level of disability.[6]
- *Pelvic floor therapy:* Essential for managing bladder and bowel dysfunction, often observed in MS patients.[7]

Occupational and Speech Therapy

- *Cognitive rehabilitation:* Addressing cognitive impairments through structured activities and exercises.[8]
- *Assistive devices:* Implementing devices to aid daily activities and enhance independence.

Integrative Health Practices

- *Yoga and Tai Chi:* Beneficial for flexibility, balance, and emotional well-being.[9,10]
- *Acupuncture:* Used for pain management and muscle spasticity, though evidence varies.

Lifestyle Interventions

Diet and Nutrition

- *Balanced diet:* Emphasis on increased fruits and vegetables, reduced processed foods, and whole grains. Specific diets such as the Mediterranean and ketogenic diets show promise in symptom management.[11]
- *Nutritional counseling:* Regular consultation with dietitians to address individual dietary needs and deficiencies.

Exercise and Physical Activity

- *Regular exercise:* Proven to reduce fatigue and improve cognitive function.[6] Recommendations include moderate aerobic exercises and strength training tailored to individual capabilities.
- *Community programs:* Participation in community-based physical activity programs enhances adherence and provides social support.

Emotional and Psychological Support

- *Counseling and therapy:* Regular sessions with mental health professionals to manage depression, anxiety, and other emotional challenges.[12]
- *Support groups*: Engagement in support groups for shared experiences and coping strategies.

SYMPTOM-BASED APPROACH TO MANAGEMENT OF SYMPTOMS IN CENTRAL NERVOUS SYSTEM DEMYELINATING DISORDERS

Fatigue

Fatigue is one of the most common and debilitating symptoms experienced by individuals with MS. It is often described as an overwhelming sense of tiredness, lack of energy, or exhaustion that is not proportional to recent activity and is not relieved by rest.

This type of fatigue can significantly impact daily functioning, reducing the quality of life and overall productivity of MS patients. Unlike normal fatigue, MS-related fatigue can occur at any time and may interfere with physical, cognitive, and emotional activities.

- *Screening method:* Fatigue severity scale (FSS), modified fatigue impact scale
- *Cutoff score:* A mean score of ≥4 in FSS indicates significant fatigue.
- *Pharmacological management:*
    - *Amantadine:* Typically 100–200 mg/day. Amantadine is a stimulant that helps reduce fatigue.[13]
    - *Modafinil:* 200 mg/day. Modafinil is a wakefulness-promoting agent that is effective in managing MS-related fatigue.

Though these drugs are given routinely for management of fatigue, they were not superior to placebo in improving MS fatigue and caused more frequent adverse events.[14]

- *Supportive measure:*
    - *Sleep hygiene education*: Educating patients on maintaining a regular sleep schedule, creating a restful environment, and avoiding stimulants before bedtime.
    - *Energy conservation techniques*: Strategies such as pacing activities, taking regular breaks, and prioritizing tasks to manage energy levels effectively.
    - *Evaluation for sleep disorders*: Conducting sleep studies to identify and treat underlying sleep disorders such as sleep apnea or restless leg syndrome.[15]

Cognitive Impairment

Cognitive impairment is a significant and often under-recognized symptom of MS, affecting approximately 40–70% of individuals with the disease. It encompasses a range of cognitive deficits that can impact memory, attention, information processing speed, executive function, and visuospatial abilities.[16] These cognitive changes can occur at any stage of the disease, even in the early relapsing-remitting phase, and can progress over time, profoundly affecting daily life, work, and social interactions.

Assessing cognitive impairment in MS is essential for developing effective management strategies. Tools such as the Symbol Digit Modalities Test (SDMT) are commonly used to screen for cognitive deficits, providing a quick and reliable measure of cognitive function.[16] Management of cognitive impairment often involves a combination of pharmacological treatments and nonpharmacological interventions, including cognitive rehabilitation, lifestyle modifications, and supportive therapies.[17]

- *Screening method:* SDMT
- *Cutoff score:* A score that is 1.5 standard deviations below the age-matched normative mean indicates significant cognitive impairment.
- *Pharmacological management*: No pharmacological agents have shown to improve cognitive impairment in MS.[17] Dalfampridine is known to improve walking in MS patients and has shown some anecdotal benefit in cognitive dysfunction.[18]
- *Supportive measure:*
    - *Cognitive rehabilitation therapy:* Cognitive rehabilitation has shown some benefit in patients with cognitive impairment in MS.[8] Structured therapy sessions to improve cognitive functions such as memory, attention, and problem-solving skills.[8]
    - *Neuropsychological evaluation*: Comprehensive assessment to identify specific cognitive deficits and tailor individualized treatment plans.
    - *Regular cognitive exercises:* Activities such as puzzles, memory games, and computer-based cognitive training programs to maintain and enhance cognitive abilities.

Pain

Pain is a prevalent and often debilitating symptom in individuals with MS, affecting up to 55% of patients at some point during their disease course. MS-related pain can manifest in various forms, including neuropathic pain, musculoskeletal pain, and spasticity-related pain, each contributing to the overall burden of the disease. The impact of pain on quality of life is profound, influencing physical functioning, emotional well-being, and daily activities.

- *Screening method:* Brief pain inventory (BPI)[19]
- *Cutoff score:* A pain severity score of ≥4 on a scale of 0–10 is considered significant.
- *Pharmacological management:* Pharmacological approaches for MS pain include anticonvulsants, antidepressants, botulinum toxin, cannabinoids, muscle relaxants, opioid analgesics, and intrathecally administered baclofen.[5] Anticonvulsants such as gabapentin and pregabalin can be tried as first line.
    - *Gabapentin:* 300–3,600 mg/day. Gabapentin is effective for neuropathic pain.
    - *Pregabalin:* 150–600 mg/day. Pregabalin is used to treat neuropathic pain and fibromyalgia.
- *Supportive measure:*
    - *Physical therapy*: Tailored exercises and modalities to manage pain and improve physical function.
    - *Acupuncture:* An integrative approach that can help reduce pain and improve quality of life.
    - *Referral to a pain management specialist*: Comprehensive pain management strategies, including interventional techniques and multidisciplinary approaches.

Bladder Dysfunction

Bladder dysfunction is a common and distressing symptom in MS, affecting approximately 80% of individuals with the disease. This dysfunction can manifest in various forms, including urgency, frequency, incontinence, and urinary retention. These symptoms result from the disruption of neural pathways that control bladder function due to demyelination and axonal damage in the CNS.[20]

The bladder dysfunctions observed in MS can be classified into two main types: Storage and emptying problems. Storage problems include symptoms such as urgency, frequency, and urge incontinence, are often caused by an overactive bladder (detrusor overactivity). Managing bladder dysfunction in MS is crucial as it significantly impacts the quality of life, leading to social embarrassment, skin problems, recurrent urinary tract infections, and even kidney damage. The Bladder Control Scale is a practical screening tool used to assess the severity of bladder symptoms and guide treatment decisions. All patients with bladder dysfunction will need a formal urological evaluation.

- *Screening method*: Bladder control scale
- *Pharmacological method:*
    - *Oxybutynin*: 5–15 mg/day. Can be used to treat urinary urgency due to detrusor overactivity.
    - *Tolterodine:* 2–4 mg/day. Tolterodine is another antimuscarinic medication effective for treating detrusor overactivity.
    - Mirabegron and solifenacin are newer drugs that can be used for overactive bladder.[21]
- *Supportive measure:*
    - *Pelvic floor physical therapy:* Exercises to strengthen the pelvic floor muscles, which can help manage urinary incontinence.[20]
    - *Scheduled voiding:* Implementing a routine for regular bladder emptying to reduce incontinence episodes.
    - *Avoidance of bladder irritants:* Reducing intake of caffeine, alcohol, and acidic foods that can exacerbate bladder symptoms.

Spasticity

Spasticity is a prevalent symptom in MS, affecting up to 80% of individuals with the disease. It is characterized by increased muscle tone, involuntary muscle contractions, stiffness, and spasms, which can lead to pain and significant impairment in mobility and daily functioning. Spasticity in MS can vary in severity and can affect any muscle group, although it is most observed in the legs.[22] Symptoms may include muscle tightness, resistance to movement, and sudden, uncontrollable muscle spasms. These symptoms can worsen with triggers such as infections, stress, fatigue, or temperature changes. Chronic spasticity can lead to muscle shortening and joint contractures, further complicating mobility and increasing the risk of falls and injuries. Managing spasticity in MS requires a comprehensive approach that includes both pharmacological treatments and nonpharmacological interventions.[22] The Modified Ashworth Scale is commonly used to assess the severity of spasticity and guide treatment decisions.

- *Pharmacological method:*
  - *Baclofen*: 10–80 mg/day. Baclofen is a muscle relaxant, effective in reducing spasticity.
  - *Tizanidine*: 2–36 mg/day. Tizanidine is another muscle relaxant, used to manage spasticity.
- *Supportive measure:*
  - *Stretching exercises*: Regular stretching routines to maintain muscle length and reduce spasticity.
  - *Physical therapy:* Customized therapy programs focusing on stretching, strengthening, and mobility exercises.
  - *Assistive devices*: Using braces, splints, or mobility aids to improve function and reduce the impact of spasticity on daily activities.
  - *Baclofen pump*: An intrathecal baclofen pump, a surgically implanted device that continuously delivers baclofen directly into the cerebrospinal fluid (CSF) around the spinal cord can be used in refractory spasticity.

Depression and Anxiety

Depression and anxiety are prevalent among individuals with MS, significantly affecting their quality of life and disease management.[23] These mood disorders can arise from the chronic stress of living with a debilitating illness, the impact of MS symptoms on daily life, and the psychological burden of managing a progressive and often unpredictable condition. The complex interplay between MS and mental health issues can create a cycle of emotional distress that exacerbates physical symptoms and impairs overall well-being.

- *Screening method*: Patient Health Questionnaire-9 (PHQ-9)/Beck's inventory
- *Pharmacological management:*
  - *Selective serotonin reuptake inhibitors*: Examples include fluoxetine (20–60 mg/day) and sertraline (50–200 mg/day).
  - *Serotonin-norepinephrine reuptake inhibitors*: Examples include venlafaxine (75–225 mg/day) and duloxetine (30–120 mg/day).
- *Supportive measure:*
  - *Cognitive behavioral therapy (CBT):* Structured therapy sessions to address negative thought patterns and behaviors.[23]
  - *Counseling:* Regular sessions with a mental health professional to provide support and coping strategies.
  - *Stress management techniques*: Practices such as mindfulness, meditation, and relaxation exercises to manage anxiety and improve emotional well-being.

CONCLUSION

Effective symptomatic management of CNS demyelination disorders requires a multifaceted approach that integrates pharmacologic, nonpharmacologic, and lifestyle interventions. Personalized care plans addressing comorbidities and utilizing evidence-based practices are essential in optimizing patient outcomes and enhancing quality of life. Ongoing research and patient education are crucial in evolving and refining these management strategies.

REFERENCES

1. Mavandadi S, Paybast S, Mirzadeh M, Mozhdehipanah H. Dalfampridine in the treatment of primary fatigue in patients with multiple sclerosis: a randomized clinical trail. Acta Neurol Belg. 2024;124(4):1289-94.
2. Cozzi FM, Zuckerman D, Sacknovitz A, Gozum N, Syal A, Danisi F, et al. (2024). Outcomes, complications, and dosing of intrathecal baclofen in the treatment of multiple sclerosis: a systematic review. [online] Available from https://thejns.org/focus/view/journals/neurosurg-focus/56/6/article-pE14.xml. [Last accessed September, 2024].
3. Stamoula E, Siafis S, Dardalas I, Ainatzoglou A, Matsas A, Athanasiadis T, et al. (2021). Antidepressants on Multiple Sclerosis: A Review of In Vitro and In Vivo Models. Front Immunol. [online] Available from https://www.frontiersin.org/journals/immunology/articles/10.3389/fimmu.2021.677879/full. [Last accessed September, 2024].
4. Nouh RA, Kamal A, Abdelnaser A. Cannabinoids and Multiple Sclerosis: A critical Analysis of therapeutic potentials and safety concerns. Pharmaceutics. 2023;15(4):1151.
5. Chisari CG, Sgarlata E, Arena S, D'Amico E, Toscano S, Patti F. An update on the pharmacological management of pain in patients with multiple sclerosis. Expert Opin Pharmacother. 2020;21(18):2249-63.
6. Proschinger S, Kuhwand P, Rademacher A, Walzik D, Warnke C, Zimmer P, et al. Fitness, physical activity, and exercise in multiple sclerosis: a systematic review on current evidence for interactions with disease activity and progression. J Neurol. 2022;269(6):2922-40.
7. Yavas I, Emuk Y, Kahraman T. Pelvic floor muscle training on urinary incontinence and sexual function in people with multiple sclerosis: A systematic review. Mult Scler Relat Disord. 2022;58:103538.
8. Brochet B. Cognitive Rehabilitation in multiple sclerosis in the period from 2013 and 2021: A narrative review. Brain Sci. 2022;12(1):55.
9. Shohani M, Kazemi F, Rahmati S, Azami M. The effect of yoga on the quality of life and fatigue in patients with multiple sclerosis: A systematic review and meta-analysis of randomized clinical trials. Complement Ther Clin Pract. 2020;39:101087.
10. Eve J. (2021). Tai Chi and mindfulness training to improve balance in people with multiple sclerosis: A Community-based intervention study. [online] Available from https://hdl.handle.net/20.500.14394/18476 [Last accessed September, 2024].
11. Stoiloudis P, Kesidou E, Bakirtzis C, Sintila SA, Konstantinidou N, Boziki M, et al. The role of diet and interventions on multiple sclerosis: A review. Nutrients. 2022;14(6):1150.
12. Morris-Bankole H, Ho AK. Psychotherapy and professional psychological support in multiple sclerosis: Uncovering patients' patterns of access and preferences. Mult Scler Relat Disord. 2023;71:104562.
13. Sadeqi Y, Baghbanian SM, Bazi A, Ghazaeian M, Fallah S. The effectiveness of amantadine and dalfampridine in improving fatigue in patients with multiple sclerosis: A randomized, double-blind, clinical trial. Curr J Neurol. 2022;21(4):211-6.
14. Nourbakhsh Revirajan N, Morris B, Cordano C, Creasman J, Manguinao M, et al. Safety and efficacy of amantadine, modafinil, and methylphenidate for fatigue in multiple sclerosis: a randomised, placebo-controlled, crossover, double-blind trial. The Lancet Neurology. 2021;20(1):P38-48.

15. Laslett LL, Honan C, Turner JA, Dagnew B, Campbell JA, Gill TK, et al. Poor sleep and multiple sclerosis: associations with symptoms of multiple sclerosis and quality of life. J Neurol Neurosurg Psychiatry. 2022;93(11):1162-5.
16. Benedict RHB, Amato MP, DeLuca J, Geurts JJG. Cognitive impairment in multiple sclerosis: clinical management, MRI, and therapeutic avenues. The Lancet Neurology. 2020;19(10):P860-71.
17. DeLuca J, Chiaravalloti ND, Sandroff BM. Treatment and management of cognitive dysfunction in patients with multiple sclerosis. Nat Rev Neurol. 2020;16(6):319-32.
18. Korsen M, Kunz R, Schminke U, Runge U, Kohlmann T, Dressel A. Dalfampridine effects on cognition, fatigue, and dexterity. Brain Behav. 2016;7(1):e00559.
19. Ehde DM, Nitsch KP, Smiley JP. Measurement characteristics and clinical utility of the Brief Pain Inventory-Short Form for individuals with multiple sclerosis. Rehabil Psychol. 2015;60(4):365-6.
20. Vecchio M, Chiaramonte R, DI Benedetto P. Management of bladder dysfunction in multiple sclerosis: a systematic review and meta-analysis of studies regarding bladder rehabilitation. Eur J Phys Rehabil Med. 2022;58(3):387-96.
21. Brucker BM, Jericevic D, Rude T, Enemchukwu E, Pape D, Rosenblum N, et al. Mirabegron versus solifenacin in multiple sclerosis patients with overactive bladder symptoms: A prospective comparative nonrandomized study. Urology. 2020;145:94-9.
22. Cameron MH, Bethoux F, Field-Fote E, Lenderking WR, Zaiser E, Cutts KN, et al. Development of an integrated conceptual model of multiple sclerosis spasticity. Disabil Rehabil. 2024;46(13):2955-65.
23. Jellinger KA. Depression and anxiety in multiple sclerosis. Review of a fatal combination. J Neural Transm (Vienna). 2024;131(8):847-69.

Index

Page number followed by *b* refer to box, *f* refer to figure, *fc* refer to flowchart, and *t* refer to table.